ON MINDFULNESS: LIVING WITH FOCUS AND INTENTION

Cat Doss-Alt, RYT-500

On Mindfulness: Living with Focus and Intention

By: Cat Doss-Alt, RYT-500

Chapter 1: What is Mindfulness?

Mindfulness is the practice of being fully present, aware, and engaged in the moment, without distraction or judgment. It is about tuning into your thoughts, feelings, and surroundings with a clear and open mind, and without the interference of habitual reactions or expectations. When you bring mindfulness into your life, you begin to experience your world with a deeper sense of clarity and appreciation.

The concept of mindfulness is simple, yet profound. It is about giving your full attention to what is happening right now, instead of being caught up in the past or worrying about the future. This act of awareness brings a sense of calm and focus, creating a more intentional and meaningful way of living.

Mindfulness: The Art of Being Present

To understand what mindfulness is, we must first understand what it means to be present. Being present means experiencing life in real-time. It means being aware of what's happening inside and around you without trying to change or manipulate it. This is not about being passive or disengaged from life, but instead fully participating in it with clarity and focus.

We all experience moments of presence, even if we don't always recognize them as such. For example, when you are deeply absorbed in a task—whether it's reading, painting, or playing a musical instrument—you might lose track of time. You are so involved in the task at hand that everything else falls away, and you are fully immersed in the moment. This state of presence is what mindfulness seeks to cultivate, but it doesn't require a specific task to be effective. You can practice mindfulness while doing anything, from walking to eating to having a conversation.

Mindfulness is not about being in a particular state of mind or achieving a particular result. Rather, it is about noticing what is happening right now, without any desire to change or judge the experience. By simply being present, you begin to cultivate a deep connection with the present moment, which allows you to live more fully.

The Components of Mindfulness

While the practice of mindfulness may seem straightforward, it involves a set of core principles that help define it as a meaningful and transformative practice. These components include awareness, attention, and acceptance.

- **Awareness**: Awareness is the foundation of mindfulness. It is the ability to notice what is happening around you and within you. Awareness allows you to observe your thoughts, feelings, physical sensations, and the environment in an unbiased way. By becoming aware of what is present in the moment, you develop a deeper understanding of your internal and external experiences.

- **Attention**: Attention is the second key element of mindfulness. It is the act of directing your focus to whatever you are experiencing. Whether you are focused on your breath, a sound, or the sensation of your feet on the ground, attention is the practice of engaging deeply with the present moment. Attention allows you to let go of distractions and remain fully engaged in the activity at hand.

- **Acceptance**: Acceptance is the third component of mindfulness. It is about embracing what is present without judgment. Often, we judge our thoughts and feelings, labeling them as good or bad. Mindfulness, however, encourages us to observe without judgment. Instead of pushing away discomfort or craving pleasure, we simply accept the experience as it is.

Acceptance creates a sense of peace and allows us to release resistance to what is happening in the moment.

Together, awareness, attention, and acceptance form the core of mindfulness practice. These elements enable us to interact with the world in a more grounded and open way, without becoming overwhelmed by our thoughts or emotions.

The Power of the Present Moment

The present moment is where life is lived. It is where all our experiences occur, whether joyful or challenging. Yet, most of us spend a significant amount of time either thinking about the past or worrying about the future. We relive old memories or fret about things that haven't even happened yet. This mental distraction often prevents us from fully experiencing life as it is.

When we bring mindfulness to our lives, we start to shift our focus from the past and future to the present. This shift can be incredibly powerful. By focusing on the present, we begin to notice the richness of our experiences. The sensations in our bodies, the sounds in our environment, the colors in our surroundings—these become more vivid when we direct our attention to them.

Mindfulness allows us to step out of the cycle of mental rumination and anxiety. Instead of being caught up in endless thoughts, we begin to experience life directly, without the filters of worry or regret. When we are truly present, we can savor the simple pleasures of life, whether it's the taste of a meal, the warmth of the sun, or the sound of a loved one's voice.

Being in the present moment can also help us break free from stress and anxiety. When we focus on the here and now, we are less likely to get lost in future-oriented thoughts or past regrets. This reduction in mental noise leads to a more peaceful and centered state of mind.

Mindfulness and Emotional Regulation

Mindfulness has the remarkable ability to help us regulate

our emotions. In our daily lives, emotions often arise quickly and can be difficult to manage. When we feel anxious, frustrated, or overwhelmed, it's easy to react impulsively, either by suppressing the emotion or acting out in frustration. Mindfulness offers a different approach: instead of reacting to emotions, we can observe them with awareness and acceptance.

When we practice mindfulness, we begin to notice the subtle ways our emotions manifest. We can feel the tension in our bodies, the quickening of our breath, or the tightening of our chest. By bringing attention to these sensations, we can catch the emotion early before it escalates into an impulsive reaction. This awareness allows us to respond more skillfully, rather than letting our emotions control us.

Mindfulness also helps us create distance between ourselves and our emotional experiences. Instead of identifying with the emotion ("I am angry" or "I am anxious"), mindfulness encourages us to observe the emotion as a temporary experience. This shift in perspective allows us to experience emotions without being consumed by them. Over time, this can lead to greater emotional resilience, as we become less reactive and more equipped to handle difficult situations.

The Benefits of Mindfulness

Mindfulness practice has been shown to provide a wide range of benefits, both mental and physical. Regular mindfulness practice helps improve focus, emotional regulation, and overall well-being.

Mental Clarity and Focus: One of the most immediate benefits of mindfulness is improved mental clarity. By training your mind to focus on the present moment, you reduce mental clutter and distractions. This heightened focus allows you to engage more deeply with tasks and make better decisions. Whether you're working, studying, or simply having a conversation, mindfulness helps you direct your attention to what is most important in the moment.

Emotional Balance: Mindfulness has a powerful effect on emotional regulation. By cultivating awareness of your emotional states and learning to accept them without judgment, you can reduce emotional reactivity. This leads to a greater sense of emotional balance and peace, even in the face of challenging situations. You can respond to stress with calmness, handle frustration with patience, and experience joy more fully.

Stress Reduction: One of the most well-known benefits of mindfulness is its ability to reduce stress. By fostering a state of awareness and presence, mindfulness helps activate the body's relaxation response, counteracting the effects of stress. Mindfulness has been shown to lower cortisol levels (the stress hormone) and improve overall well-being. It helps us respond to stress with greater ease, rather than getting overwhelmed by it.

Improved Well-being: Mindfulness enhances overall physical and mental health. It has been linked to reduced symptoms of depression and anxiety, improved sleep, and a stronger immune system. Through the consistent practice of mindfulness, we can experience a deeper sense of joy and contentment in our lives. It helps us connect to the richness of our experiences, cultivating a greater sense of gratitude and fulfillment.

Mindfulness as a Way of Living

While mindfulness is often practiced through formal meditation, it is not confined to the cushion or a specific practice. It is a way of living that can be incorporated into every aspect of your life. Whether you are eating, walking, driving, or having a conversation, you can practice mindfulness by being present and fully engaged in the moment.

The beauty of mindfulness is that it can be practiced anywhere, at any time. It doesn't require special circumstances or equipment—it only requires a willingness to pay attention and be present. The more you practice, the more natural it becomes to engage mindfully with your experiences.

When mindfulness becomes a way of living, it transforms your relationship with the world. You become more attuned to the subtleties of life—the smells, sounds, and sensations that often go unnoticed. Your relationships deepen as you learn to be fully present with others, listening attentively and responding with empathy. You begin to live with greater intention, choosing your actions, thoughts, and words based on what matters most to you.

Living With Intention

Mindfulness is not just a practice; it is a way of living more fully and more intentionally. By bringing awareness, attention, and acceptance into our daily lives, we can transform our experience of the world. Mindfulness allows us to step out of the automatic patterns of behavior and engage with life as it is, with clarity, focus, and compassion.

As you begin to explore mindfulness, remember that it is not about striving for perfection. It's about being present with whatever arises, accepting each moment as it is, and living with greater awareness and intention. With regular practice, mindfulness will become a natural part of your life, helping you cultivate peace, clarity, and well-being.

CHAPTER 2: THE PRACTICAL BENEFITS OF MINDFULNESS

Mindfulness is not just a concept reserved for meditation practitioners or spiritual seekers. It is a practical tool that can bring tangible benefits to all areas of life. From boosting emotional resilience to enhancing physical health and improving relationships, mindfulness offers powerful ways to enrich our experiences, increase productivity, and foster well-being. This chapter explores the wide-ranging benefits of mindfulness, demonstrating how it can profoundly transform the way we think, feel, and interact with others.

How Mindfulness Improves Daily Life

Mindfulness is not just a mental exercise—it's a way of living that can profoundly enhance your daily life. At its core, mindfulness involves being present and engaged in the moment, which allows you to experience life more fully. Whether it's a busy day at work, a quiet moment at home, or a social gathering, mindfulness offers a way to navigate everyday situations with greater clarity, calmness, and intention.

One of the most powerful ways that mindfulness improves daily life is by helping you better manage your thoughts, emotions, and actions. Often, we react to situations automatically—responding to stress with frustration, feeling overwhelmed by distractions, or becoming caught in negative thinking patterns. Mindfulness gives you the ability to pause, observe, and respond more thoughtfully rather than react impulsively. This simple shift leads to greater emotional regulation and resilience, helping you maintain a sense of calm even in challenging situations.

For example, when dealing with a stressful project at work, mindfulness helps you stay focused and grounded. Instead of allowing frustration to cloud your thoughts, mindfulness helps you stay connected to the present moment. It encourages you to take short breaks, breathe deeply, and refocus on the task at hand. This increased mental clarity and emotional regulation leads to more effective decision-making, reduced stress, and a sense of accomplishment as you move through your day.

By cultivating mindfulness, you learn to engage with each moment without judgment. You experience life as it happens, without getting lost in the past or worrying about the future. This awareness of the present helps you feel more alive, improving the quality of your experience and deepening your connection to the world around you.

Mindfulness and the Body

Mindfulness does more than improve mental clarity and emotional resilience; it also has significant benefits for the body. The mind and body are intimately connected, and the way we think and feel can directly impact our physical health. When we practice mindfulness, we cultivate a state of awareness that reduces stress, improves sleep, and supports overall vitality.

One of the key ways mindfulness promotes physical health is by reducing stress. Chronic stress has been shown to negatively affect almost every system in the body, from the immune system to the cardiovascular system. Stress can increase the risk of developing conditions such as heart disease, high blood pressure, and diabetes. It can also weaken the immune system, making us more susceptible to illness.

Mindfulness helps counteract the effects of stress by activating the body's relaxation response. This physiological process reduces the production of stress hormones, such as cortisol, and encourages a state of calm. When practiced regularly, mindfulness helps lower overall stress levels, improving long-term health outcomes. By learning to manage stress through mindfulness, we can prevent the physical toll it takes on the body.

In addition to reducing stress, mindfulness improves sleep. Many people struggle with sleep-related issues, such as insomnia, due to stress, anxiety, or racing thoughts. Mindfulness can help break this cycle by promoting relaxation and quieting the mind. Mindfulness techniques, such as deep breathing and body scanning, can help you unwind before bed, allowing you to fall asleep more easily and experience a deeper, more restorative rest. This improvement in sleep quality leads to greater energy, improved mood, and better overall health.

Mindfulness also supports overall vitality by fostering a greater awareness of the body. When we are distracted or disconnected from our physical sensations, we may overlook important signals our body is sending. Mindfulness encourages us to pay attention to how we feel physically—whether it's hunger, tension, or fatigue—allowing us to respond with more care. This awareness helps promote healthier habits, such as eating mindfully, moving the body more, and practicing self-care, all of which contribute to long-term vitality.

Mindfulness in Overcoming Negative States

Negative emotional states, such as anxiety, anger, frustration, and sadness, are part of the human experience. These emotions can arise at any time, and when left unchecked, they can lead to greater stress, conflict, and unhappiness. Fortunately, mindfulness offers powerful tools for managing and transforming these negative states.

One of the ways mindfulness helps with negative emotions is by encouraging us to observe them without judgment. Often, when we experience intense emotions, we try to suppress or deny them. This avoidance creates internal tension, making the emotions even harder to manage. Mindfulness, however, teaches us to sit with emotions as they arise and observe them with awareness and acceptance. Rather than labeling the emotion as "good" or "bad," we learn to see it as a temporary experience that will eventually pass.

For example, when anxiety arises, mindfulness allows us to acknowledge the feeling without becoming consumed by it. We might notice the tightness in our chest or the rapidity of our breath, but we don't judge ourselves for feeling anxious. Instead, we simply observe the sensation with curiosity and compassion. This non-reactive awareness helps us create space between ourselves and the emotion, reducing its intensity and allowing us to respond more skillfully.

Mindfulness also encourages the development of self-compassion, which is key to overcoming negative emotional states. Instead of criticizing ourselves for feeling anxious, angry, or frustrated, mindfulness teaches us to be kind and understanding toward ourselves. We may say to ourselves, "It's okay to feel this way. I'm doing the best I can." This self-compassionate mindset helps us navigate negative emotions with greater ease, without becoming overwhelmed or self-critical.

Over time, practicing mindfulness helps us develop emotional awareness, which enables us to recognize patterns in our emotional responses. As we become more attuned to our emotional states, we can identify triggers and choose more constructive ways to deal with them. By developing a mindful approach to our emotions, we are better equipped to manage difficult feelings and prevent them from spiraling out of control.

Mindfulness and Performance

Mindfulness is not just about emotional regulation; it also has a profound impact on performance. Whether in the workplace, in creative endeavors, or in personal goals, mindfulness enhances productivity, creativity, and decision-making. By cultivating focus and clarity, mindfulness helps you perform at your best, without being bogged down by distractions or stress.

One of the ways mindfulness boosts performance is by enhancing concentration and focus. In our busy, fast-paced lives, it's easy to become distracted by external stimuli or our own racing thoughts. Mindfulness helps sharpen our focus by training the mind to stay present in the moment. When we bring our attention fully to the task at hand, we become more efficient and effective in our work. Whether you're writing, solving a problem, or engaging in a conversation, mindfulness allows you to stay fully engaged and produce higher-quality results.

In addition to improving focus, mindfulness enhances creativity by fostering a calm and open mind. Creativity thrives in an environment free from judgment and stress. Mindfulness helps clear mental clutter, making space for new ideas to emerge. By practicing mindfulness, you become more attuned to your inner creativity, allowing you to approach challenges with fresh perspectives and innovative solutions.

Mindfulness also improves decision-making by promoting clarity and awareness. In moments of decision, we often feel pressured to make quick choices or become overwhelmed by the options available. Mindfulness allows us to slow down, observe our thoughts and feelings, and make decisions that are aligned with our values and goals. This mindful approach leads to better decision-making, as we are able to make choices that serve our long-term well-being, rather than reacting impulsively or out of fear.

Mindfulness and Social Connections

One of the most profound benefits of mindfulness is its ability to improve relationships. By fostering presence, empathy, and compassion, mindfulness helps us connect more deeply with others, creating stronger and more meaningful social bonds.

Mindfulness helps improve communication by encouraging active listening. In our fast-paced world, we often listen to others with the intent of responding, rather than truly hearing what they are saying. Mindfulness shifts this dynamic by teaching us to listen with full attention. We become more present with the speaker, noticing their words, tone, and body language. This deep listening fosters greater understanding and connection, allowing us to respond with empathy and compassion.

In addition to enhancing communication, mindfulness helps us develop greater empathy. By being present with our own emotions, we become more attuned to the emotions of others. We are able to recognize their feelings, even if they are not explicitly expressed, and respond in ways that are supportive and caring. Mindfulness also encourages non-judgment, which helps us accept others as they are, without trying to change or criticize them.

Mindfulness plays a crucial role in conflict resolution by allowing us to approach disagreements with a calm and open mind. Instead of reacting impulsively to a disagreement, mindfulness encourages us to pause, take a deep breath, and consider the other person's perspective. This mindful approach helps create space for constructive dialogue and problem-solving, reducing the likelihood of escalating conflicts.

Mindfulness as a Transformative Tool

Mindfulness is a transformative tool that brings tangible benefits to the mind, body, and relationships. By improving emotional regulation, enhancing physical health, boosting performance, and fostering deeper connections with others, mindfulness helps us live more fulfilling and meaningful lives. It is not just a practice but a way of being—one that allows us to approach life with greater clarity, compassion, and resilience.

Whether you're looking to manage stress, improve your health, boost your productivity, or enhance your relationships, mindfulness provides the tools to create lasting positive change. As you continue to integrate mindfulness into your life, you will discover its many benefits and experience the profound impact it can have on your overall well-being.

CHAPTER 3: THE POWER OF THE PRESENT MOMENT

The present moment is often overlooked, yet it holds incredible power. We tend to focus on the past or the future, but it is the present that shapes our experiences, our thoughts, and our emotions. When we are fully engaged with the here and now, we unlock the potential for deeper clarity, reduced anxiety, and more meaningful experiences. This chapter explores the significance of the present moment, how our minds tend to wander, and how we can cultivate a greater awareness of the present.

The Importance of Being Present

At its core, mindfulness is about being fully present in the moment. In a world that is often filled with distractions, being present is more difficult than it seems, yet it is the key to unlocking a life of greater clarity, peace, and fulfillment. When we are present, we experience life directly. We engage with our surroundings, our relationships, and our thoughts with full attention and awareness. This allows us to make conscious choices, deepen our connections with others, and gain a greater understanding of ourselves.

Being present is not just about physical presence—it's about mental presence as well. It means fully immersing yourself in whatever you're doing, without being distracted by your thoughts, worries, or to-do lists. Whether you're having a conversation, working on a project, or simply enjoying a meal, the more present you are, the more enriching the experience becomes.

When we are fully present, we are less likely to get caught up in the "shoulds" of life—the constant pressure to do more, be more, and achieve more. Instead of feeling like we are running on autopilot, we are actively participating in life. This sense of presence leads to greater contentment and satisfaction. We begin to realize that the present moment is the only time that is truly ours. The past is gone, and the future is unknown, but the present is where life is happening.

How Our Minds Wander: The Toll of Past and Future Thinking

While the present moment is powerful, it is often elusive. Our minds have a tendency to wander—often to the past or the future. This is a natural part of being human, but when we spend too much time dwelling on the past or worrying about the future, it can take a toll on our mental health.

When we focus on the past, we may replay old conversations or experiences, replaying moments of regret, shame, or anger. These memories, whether positive or negative, can prevent us from fully engaging with the present. We may find ourselves ruminating over past mistakes or wishing we could go back and do things differently. While reflection can be helpful in learning from the past, excessive dwelling on what has already happened prevents us from experiencing the present moment fully.

Similarly, when we focus too much on the future, we may become anxious about what might happen. We worry about things that are outside our control, creating a sense of unease. The future, unlike the past, is unknown, and our imaginations often run wild with possibilities. We may worry about potential outcomes, about whether we'll succeed or fail, or about what others will think of us. This constant future-focused thinking creates stress and uncertainty, stealing our peace in the present.

The toll of past and future thinking is clear. Our attention becomes divided, our minds cluttered, and our emotional state is influenced by thoughts of what is not real or no longer relevant. The result is a feeling of disconnection—from ourselves, from others, and from the world around us. We miss out on the richness of the present moment, focusing instead on the fleeting nature of time. And the more we dwell in these thoughts, the more stress, anxiety, and frustration accumulate.

But there is good news: the practice of mindfulness offers a way to break free from this cycle of distraction. By training ourselves to focus on the present, we can reduce the power that past and future thinking has over us. We can begin to reclaim our mental energy and experience life as it happens, in all its richness and complexity.

The Mental Toll of Distraction

The constant mental distractions caused by past and future thinking have been shown to have negative effects on our mental and emotional well-being. Studies have found that people who spend more time thinking about the past or future tend to experience higher levels of stress and anxiety. This is because the mind is constantly running through scenarios—both real and imagined—that induce tension.

When we worry about the future, our minds create stories, often filled with worst-case scenarios. These stories trigger the body's stress response, causing an increase in heart rate, shallow breathing, and muscle tension. This stress response can become chronic if we are consistently focused on what might go wrong, rather than what is happening in the present.

Similarly, when we dwell on the past, we may revisit painful memories, old wounds, or missed opportunities. This can trigger emotions like sadness, guilt, or regret. These emotions, while valid, often keep us stuck in a cycle of negative thinking, preventing us from moving forward and fully engaging with life as it is now.

The act of multitasking—constantly switching between tasks

and trying to keep track of multiple things at once—can further fragment our attention and exacerbate these mental strains. Research has shown that multitasking actually reduces productivity and increases cognitive load. When we are constantly shifting between tasks or thoughts, our mental resources are stretched thin, leaving us mentally exhausted.

Being mindful of the present moment is a powerful antidote to this constant distraction. By focusing on one thing at a time and bringing our attention back to the here and now, we can train our brains to be more resilient, centered, and clear.

Techniques for Cultivating Awareness of the Present Moment

Cultivating present-moment awareness is a skill that can be developed with consistent practice. There are several techniques that can help you stay connected to the present, no matter what you're doing. These practices encourage a mindful approach to everyday life, helping you break free from the cycle of distraction and mental clutter.

1. **Mindful Breathing:** One of the simplest ways to return to the present moment is by focusing on your breath. Pay attention to the sensation of the air entering and leaving your body. Notice the rise and fall of your chest or abdomen with each breath. When your mind begins to wander, gently bring your focus back to the breath. This practice helps anchor your attention to the present and can be done anywhere—at your desk, in the car, or even during a conversation.

2. **Body Scan:** A body scan is a technique where you focus your attention on each part of your body, starting from the top of your head and working your way down to your toes. As you do so, notice any sensations, tensions, or areas of discomfort. This practice helps you reconnect with your body and brings your awareness into the present moment. It is particularly useful for grounding yourself when you

feel disconnected or distracted.

3. **Mindful Listening:** Another technique to stay present is mindful listening. In conversations, instead of planning your next response or thinking about what you want to say, focus entirely on the speaker. Pay attention to their words, tone, and body language. Listen without judgment or interruption. This practice not only helps you stay present but also improves your communication and relationships with others.

4. **Engaging the Senses:** Using your senses is a powerful way to anchor yourself in the present moment. Notice the colors, textures, and smells around you. Feel the sensation of your feet on the ground or the warmth of the sun on your skin. Engaging the senses draws your attention to what is happening right now, shifting your focus away from distracting thoughts.

5. **Mindful Movement:** Mindfulness doesn't just apply to stillness—it can also be incorporated into movement. Whether you're walking, running, or doing yoga, try to bring your full attention to the sensations of movement. Feel the rhythm of your body, the ground beneath your feet, and the breath as it moves through you. This practice helps create a sense of flow and connection with your body.

6. **Journaling:** Writing down your thoughts and feelings can be an effective way to anchor yourself in the present. Journaling allows you to express your emotions and process your experiences in real-time. It also helps clear mental clutter and create space for greater awareness.

By incorporating these techniques into your daily life, you can strengthen your ability to stay present and reduce the mental distractions that pull you away from the here and now. Over time, these practices become second nature, and you will find it easier to be fully engaged with whatever you are doing, no matter how mundane or challenging.

Being Present: The Key to Reducing Anxiety and Enhancing Our Experience of Life

The power of the present moment is immense. By cultivating awareness of the here and now, we can reduce the mental toll of past and future thinking and enhance our overall experience of life. Being present helps us become more grounded, more focused, and more connected to ourselves and others. It allows us to experience life as it unfolds, rather than getting caught up in distractions or worries.

When we learn to focus on the present moment, we reduce anxiety and stress, improve emotional regulation, and increase our ability to handle challenges. Mindfulness offers a way to reclaim our attention, break free from negative thought patterns, and experience a greater sense of peace and fulfillment.

The present moment is all we have, and when we learn to fully inhabit it, we open ourselves up to a life of deeper joy, meaning, and connection. By practicing mindfulness, we can make the most of each moment, and in doing so, transform our experience of life.

Mindful Living: Focus and Wellbeing in Everyday Life

CHAPTER 4: MINDFULNESS AND STRESS RELIEF

Stress is a ubiquitous part of life, affecting nearly everyone in some form or another. From the pressures of responsibilities to the challenges of daily life, stress can be overwhelming and, if left unchecked, can have serious consequences for both our mental and physical health. However, mindfulness offers a powerful tool to manage and reduce stress. By cultivating a state of present-moment awareness, mindfulness helps us break free from the automatic reactions that stress often triggers, allowing us to respond more calmly, thoughtfully, and with greater resilience.

In this chapter, we will explore how stress affects both the body and the mind, why mindfulness is such an effective antidote, the role of breath in managing stress, and how to incorporate mindful awareness into stressful situations. By the end of this chapter, you will understand how mindfulness can transform your relationship with stress and provide you with a set of practical tools to stay calm and centered, even in the most challenging situations.

How Stress Affects the Body and Mind

Before we explore how mindfulness can relieve stress, it is important to understand how stress affects us physically and emotionally. Stress is the body's natural response to a perceived threat or challenge. This response is known as the "fight or flight" reaction, a mechanism that has evolved to help us survive dangerous situations.

When the body perceives a threat, the brain signals the release of stress hormones like cortisol and adrenaline. These hormones prepare the body to take action—whether that means fighting the threat or fleeing from it. In the short term, this stress response is essential for survival. However, when stress is chronic or prolonged, it can have harmful effects on both our physical and mental health.

Physically, prolonged stress can lead to a range of health problems, including headaches, muscle tension, high blood pressure, digestive issues, and weakened immune function. It can also contribute to more serious conditions like heart disease, diabetes, and chronic fatigue.

Emotionally, stress can lead to feelings of anxiety, irritability, and overwhelm. The constant state of heightened alertness that comes with stress can make it difficult to relax or think clearly. This can negatively impact our ability to make decisions, communicate effectively, or perform tasks efficiently. Over time, chronic stress can contribute to mental health issues like depression and anxiety disorders.

Mindfulness provides an antidote to these harmful effects of stress by helping us break free from the cycle of constant reactivity. Instead of reacting automatically to stressors, mindfulness encourages us to pause, observe our thoughts and feelings, and respond in a more thoughtful and measured way. This can reduce the physiological and psychological toll of stress and help us regain a sense of calm and control.

Why Mindfulness is Effective for Stress Relief

Mindfulness is particularly effective for managing stress because it works by directly counteracting the body's natural stress response. In a stressful situation, the body automatically shifts into a state of heightened alertness, preparing us for fight or flight. However, when we practice mindfulness, we consciously activate the body's relaxation response, which is the opposite of the stress response.

The relaxation response was first coined by Dr. Herbert Benson in the 1970s. It refers to the physiological state that occurs when the body experiences a reduction in stress hormones, heart rate, and blood pressure. This state promotes relaxation and a sense of calm, allowing the body to recover from the effects of stress.

Mindfulness encourages the relaxation response by helping us focus on the present moment, rather than getting caught up in the worries and anxieties that often accompany stressful situations. When we are mindful, we direct our attention away from thoughts about the future or the past and instead focus on our immediate experience. This shift in focus can help calm the nervous system, lower cortisol levels, and create a sense of ease in the body and mind.

Research has shown that regular mindfulness practice can reduce the body's overall stress response. Studies have demonstrated that individuals who practice mindfulness have lower levels of cortisol and report feeling less stressed in their daily lives. Mindfulness also helps us become more resilient to stress by teaching us how to respond to challenges with a sense of calm and clarity, rather than reacting impulsively or becoming overwhelmed.

In addition to reducing the physiological effects of stress, mindfulness also helps improve emotional regulation. When we are mindful, we learn to observe our emotions without becoming consumed by them. This allows us to acknowledge and process our feelings of stress without letting them control our behavior or well-being.

The Role of Breath in Calming the Nervous System

One of the most powerful tools we have for managing stress is the breath. When we are stressed, our breathing becomes shallow and rapid. This activates the body's stress response, increasing tension and discomfort. On the other hand, when we focus on slow, deep breathing, we can activate the body's relaxation response, calming the nervous system and promoting a sense of peace.

The breath is a natural and immediate way to bring mindfulness into our daily lives. By paying attention to the breath, we can interrupt the cycle of stress and bring ourselves back to the present moment. Deep breathing not only calms the body but also creates a mental shift. It signals to the brain that we are safe and that there is no immediate threat.

There are several types of breathing techniques that can help manage stress and activate the relaxation response. One of the most well-known techniques is diaphragmatic breathing, also known as abdominal or belly breathing. To practice diaphragmatic breathing, place one hand on your chest and the other on your abdomen. As you breathe in, allow your abdomen to rise, filling your lungs with air. As you breathe out, allow your abdomen to fall. This type of deep breathing engages the diaphragm, allowing for a full breath that relaxes the body and calms the mind.

Another effective breathing technique is known as 4-7-8 breathing. To practice this technique, inhale quietly through your nose for a count of four, hold your breath for a count of seven, and exhale completely through your mouth for a count of eight. This technique helps slow down the breath, which in turn activates the parasympathetic nervous system and induces a state of calm.

By incorporating these breathing techniques into your daily routine, you can learn to manage stress more effectively and prevent the physical and emotional toll that stress can take on the body and mind.

Mindful Awareness in Managing Stressful Situations

In addition to using breathwork to calm the body, mindfulness also encourages a shift in how we approach stressful situations. Rather than avoiding or fighting stress, mindfulness invites us to face it head-on with openness and curiosity. This does not mean that stress will magically disappear, but it does mean that we can change our relationship with it.

One key aspect of mindful stress management is cultivating awareness of the present moment. In stressful situations, our minds often race, jumping from one thought to the next, creating a cycle of worry and anxiety. Mindfulness teaches us to pause and notice these thoughts as they arise, without judgment. By observing our thoughts and feelings with curiosity, we create a space between ourselves and the stress, which allows us to respond more thoughtfully.

For example, if you are in a meeting and feeling overwhelmed, mindfulness allows you to acknowledge the feeling of stress without letting it take over. Rather than getting caught up in negative self-talk or worrying about the outcome, you can focus on your breath, bring your attention to the present moment, and approach the situation with a clearer, calmer mind. This shift in awareness can help you navigate challenging situations with greater ease and confidence.

Mindfulness also encourages us to be more accepting of stress, rather than trying to eliminate it altogether. Stress is a natural part of life, and by acknowledging it without resistance, we can reduce its intensity. When we resist stress or try to fight it, we only amplify its effects. However, when we accept stress as a temporary and normal part of our experience, we are better able to deal with it in a balanced way.

Another important aspect of mindful awareness is recognizing the impact of stress on the body. Stress often manifests physically in the form of muscle tension, headaches, or tightness in the chest. By practicing mindfulness, we become more attuned to these physical sensations and can use them as cues to slow down and take care of ourselves. For instance, if you notice that you are clenching your jaw or tensing your shoulders, you can consciously release that tension and take a few deep breaths.

This mindful awareness of the body helps us prevent stress from accumulating and becoming overwhelming.

Practical Techniques for Managing Stress Mindfully

1. **Mindful Walking:** Walking mindfully involves paying full attention to the sensation of movement as you walk. Focus on the feel of your feet on the ground, the rhythm of your steps, and the environment around you. This practice can help you take a break from stressful thoughts and reconnect with the present moment.

2. **Mindful Pauses:** Throughout the day, take short mindful pauses to check in with yourself. This could be as simple as taking a few deep breaths or pausing for a moment of reflection. These brief moments of mindfulness can help you stay grounded and reduce stress before it builds up.

3. **Mindful Listening:** When in a stressful conversation, practice mindful listening by focusing entirely on the speaker without judgment or distraction. This helps you stay present in the moment and reduces the emotional charge of the interaction.

Mindfulness Helps Us Stay Calm and Centered, Even Under Pressure

Mindfulness is a powerful tool for managing and relieving stress. By cultivating awareness of the present moment, practicing deep breathing, and responding to stressful situations with openness and acceptance, we can reduce the impact of stress on our bodies and minds. Mindfulness allows us to stay calm and centered, even in the most challenging circumstances, and empowers us to approach stress with greater clarity, resilience, and compassion.

Through regular mindfulness practice, we can transform our relationship with stress, promoting emotional regulation, enhancing our ability to cope with difficulties, and improving our overall well-being.

CHAPTER 5: BUILDING A MINDFUL FOUNDATION

Mindfulness is more than just a practice—it is a way of living. It's about being present and aware in every moment, bringing a sense of focus and clarity to the ordinary aspects of our day-to-day lives. For many, the idea of mindfulness is often reserved for moments of meditation or stillness. However, to truly benefit from mindfulness, it must be integrated into the fabric of everyday life. The goal is not just to practice mindfulness for a few minutes each day but to build a foundation of mindful living that shapes your entire approach to life.

In this chapter, we will explore how to start integrating mindfulness into your daily routine, providing simple and effective practices that you can adopt to cultivate mindfulness throughout the day. We will also discuss the importance of consistency in building a sustainable practice, and how making mindfulness a habit can lead to lasting wellbeing.

How to Start Integrating Mindfulness into Your Daily Life

Building a mindful foundation begins with the decision to make mindfulness a part of your life, rather than just an activity. It's about shifting your mindset to prioritize awareness and presence. This shift doesn't require grand gestures or dramatic changes—what matters is the small, consistent steps you take to bring mindfulness into the moment.

One of the easiest ways to integrate mindfulness into your daily life is by starting with your breath. The breath is always present, always with you, and it provides a direct gateway into the present moment. Bringing awareness to your breath throughout the day, even for just a few moments, is a powerful way to anchor yourself in the here and now.

Begin by setting aside a few minutes each day for mindful breathing. This can be as simple as taking a few deep breaths while sitting quietly at the start or end of your day. Focus all your attention on the sensation of the breath entering and leaving your body. When your mind inevitably starts to wander, gently bring your attention back to the breath, noticing the rise and fall of your chest or abdomen with each inhale and exhale. This practice is not about forcing your thoughts to stop, but rather about training your mind to return to the present moment.

Another way to start integrating mindfulness is by performing simple tasks with full attention. For example, washing dishes, brushing your teeth, or walking to work are all opportunities to practice mindfulness. Instead of rushing through these activities while your mind races ahead, focus entirely on the task at hand. Notice the textures, sounds, and sensations involved. If you're washing dishes, feel the warmth of the water, hear the clink of the plates, and observe the movements of your hands. This practice, often called "mindful doing," helps you bring the same level of attention to the smallest activities as you would in a formal meditation session.

As you begin to integrate mindfulness into your day, it's essential to recognize that the goal is not perfection, but awareness. The more you practice being present in everyday activities, the more natural it will become to bring mindfulness into all areas of your life.

Simple Practices for Cultivating Mindfulness in Routine Activities

One of the most effective ways to build a mindful foundation is to incorporate mindfulness into routine activities. When practiced consistently, these small actions can create a steady stream of mindful moments throughout the day, making it easier to maintain a sense of calm and clarity.

1. Mindful Walking: Walking is another routine activity that offers numerous opportunities for mindfulness. Whether you are walking to work, walking the dog, or simply moving from one room to another, you can use each step as a reminder to return to the present moment. As you walk, notice the sensation of your feet touching the ground, the rhythm of your steps, and the movement of your body. Be aware of your surroundings —the sounds, the sights, and the air you breathe. Walking mindfully is a simple but powerful way to bring more awareness into your day.

2. Mindful Listening: We spend much of our time listening to others, yet we are often distracted by our own thoughts and judgments. Mindful listening is about truly being present when someone is speaking, without interrupting, planning your response, or drifting into your own thoughts. When you listen mindfully, you give your full attention to the speaker, noticing the tone of their voice, their body language, and the words they use. This practice not only strengthens your ability to focus but also enhances your relationships by making others feel heard and understood.

3. Mindful Breathing During Transitions: Transitions between activities can be stressful or hurried, often leading to a scattered state of mind. However, you can use transitions as opportunities to practice mindfulness. Whether you are moving from one meeting to another, switching tasks, or simply going from one room to another, take a moment to pause and breathe. Close your eyes for a second, take a deep breath, and center yourself before moving on. This brief pause will help you reset your mind and approach the next activity with greater focus and clarity.

4. Mindful Technology Use: In today's world, we are constantly surrounded by technology, from smartphones and computers to social media and emails. Technology can often be a source of stress and distraction. To practice mindfulness with technology, try to bring more awareness to how and when you use your devices. Set boundaries around your screen time, and when you are using technology, do so with intention. Rather than mindlessly scrolling or checking your phone every few minutes, take time to notice your thoughts and feelings as you interact with your devices. When you're done, try to fully disengage rather than letting your attention stay split. This mindful approach to technology can reduce the overwhelm often associated with constant connectivity.

The Importance of Consistency in Building a Sustainable Mindfulness Practice

One of the most important aspects of building a mindful foundation is consistency. While occasional mindfulness practice can be beneficial, regular, consistent practice is key to experiencing lasting changes in your life. Just as physical exercise strengthens your muscles over time, mindfulness strengthens your ability to focus, regulate your emotions, and respond to stress more effectively. But like any skill, mindfulness requires practice.

To build a sustainable mindfulness practice, it's essential to start small and be consistent. Begin by committing to just a few minutes of mindfulness each day, and gradually increase the amount of time you dedicate to the practice as it becomes a more natural part of your routine. Consistency is more important than duration. Practicing for five minutes each day is more beneficial than practicing for an hour once a week.

One way to cultivate consistency is by anchoring your mindfulness practice to an existing habit. For example, you might decide to practice mindful breathing every time you sit down for a meal or take a mindful pause whenever you wake up in the morning. By tying mindfulness to an established routine, you create a seamless transition between your daily activities and your mindfulness practice.

Another important aspect of consistency is developing a mindset of patience and self-compassion. It's easy to become frustrated if you don't feel the benefits of mindfulness right away, but mindfulness is a long-term practice. Just as physical fitness doesn't happen overnight, neither does mental and emotional fitness. It takes time to train the mind to be more present and focused. Be kind to yourself, and remember that every moment of mindfulness is valuable, even if it feels fleeting or difficult at first.

Overcoming Challenges in Maintaining a Mindful Practice

While mindfulness offers many benefits, building a consistent practice isn't always easy. Life can get in the way, distractions can arise, and old habits can be hard to break. However, acknowledging these challenges is an important part of the process. Here are some strategies to overcome common obstacles in maintaining a consistent mindfulness practice:

1. **Set Realistic Expectations:** Start with small, achievable goals. Don't overwhelm yourself by trying to commit to long meditation sessions or a rigorous routine right away. Even five minutes of mindfulness can be powerful, especially when practiced regularly.

2. **Make Mindfulness Enjoyable:** Find ways to make mindfulness enjoyable and meaningful for you. If you enjoy being outdoors, take your mindfulness practice to the park or go for a mindful walk. If you love food, try mindful eating. The more enjoyable your practice is, the more likely you are to stick with it.

3. **Create a Supportive Environment:** Surround yourself with reminders and tools that encourage mindfulness. Set aside a designated time and space for practice, and consider using mindfulness apps or journals to track your progress. Having a supportive environment makes it easier to stay consistent.

4. Be Patient with Yourself: It's normal for your mind to wander during mindfulness practice. The key is to notice when it happens and gently bring your focus back. Don't judge yourself for losing focus—this is part of the practice. Mindfulness is not about achieving perfection, but about being present with whatever arises.

Consistent Mindfulness Builds a Foundation for Lasting Wellbeing

The foundation of mindfulness is built on small, consistent actions that, over time, lead to profound changes in how we experience life. By integrating mindfulness into everyday activities, cultivating regular practice, and being patient with ourselves, we create a foundation of awareness, presence, and calm that supports lasting wellbeing.

Mindfulness is not a quick fix or a one-time solution to stress and distraction. It is a lifelong practice that can enhance every aspect of our lives—our health, our relationships, our work, and our inner peace. As you begin to build your own mindful foundation, remember that the key to success lies in consistency. By practicing mindfulness daily, you will gradually notice its positive impact, helping you live with greater clarity, balance, and joy.

CHAPTER 6 : CREATING A PEACEFUL SPACE

In a world that can often feel overwhelming, a peaceful environment at home serves as a sanctuary—a place where you can retreat, find calm, and replenish your energy. Creating a mindful space in your home is about more than just physical appearance; it's about curating an atmosphere that supports your mental well-being and encourages tranquility. Whether it's a quiet corner for reflection, a cozy reading nook, or simply the overall energy of your living space, the goal is to create an environment where mindfulness can flourish.

This chapter explores how to design a space that promotes relaxation, focus, and emotional balance. The essence of a peaceful home is rooted in both physical and emotional simplicity—less clutter, more clarity, and intentional surroundings that help you stay grounded and present. In the following pages, we'll explore how to achieve this balance by focusing on sensory experiences, organization, and creating an intentional ambiance.

The Power of Space

The spaces we inhabit have a direct impact on our mental and emotional state. Our surroundings affect the way we feel, behave, and interact with the world around us. A cluttered or chaotic environment can heighten stress, distraction, and unease. On the other hand, a well-organized, serene environment can foster relaxation, mental clarity, and emotional balance. By intentionally crafting a space that aligns with your values, desires, and emotional needs, you can nurture a sense of well-being that supports mindfulness throughout your daily life.

The first step in creating a peaceful space is recognizing the importance of intentionality. A peaceful environment doesn't happen by accident—it's the result of thoughtful decisions made with your mental and emotional health in mind. A mindful space is free of distractions and clutter, but it's also one that brings you comfort, inspiration, and calm.

Decluttering: Simplifying for Clarity

One of the first steps to creating a peaceful home is decluttering. In a space filled with excess, it's difficult to focus or unwind. Clutter can cloud your thoughts and make it harder to be present. Decluttering isn't just about tidying up; it's about clearing out what no longer serves you, both physically and emotionally. This could mean letting go of items that no longer hold value or repurposing spaces that aren't being used effectively.

Start by evaluating each room in your home. Do you feel calm when you walk into them, or do you feel overwhelmed by the amount of stuff? Begin with one space at a time, whether it's a single room or even a small corner. Choose what to keep by considering what sparks joy, brings utility, or promotes relaxation. This might mean keeping only the items you truly need or cherish, from furniture to decorative pieces.

In addition to clearing away unnecessary items, organizing your space in a functional way also contributes to a peaceful environment. Store things out of sight to keep surfaces clear and allow for easy access to the items you do use regularly. Make sure everything has its place, and try to maintain that order over time.

Sensory Design: Tuning Into Your Senses

A peaceful space engages all of the senses. The physical environment is more than just a visual experience; it's about how a room feels, smells, sounds, and even tastes. Mindfully incorporating sensory elements into your space can elevate the sense of calm and help you feel present in the moment.

- **Sight**: Start by thinking about the color scheme of your space. Colors have a significant impact on how we feel. Soft, neutral tones such as whites, beige, and pastels can promote calmness, while deeper tones like navy or forest green may evoke a sense of groundedness. To make the space feel more open and serene, opt for natural light when possible, and use light-colored furniture and soft textures. Minimalism is often an effective approach here, as it eliminates distractions and allows you to focus on the beauty of simple, clean lines.

- **Sound**: Silence can be golden, but ambient sound can also contribute to a peaceful environment. Subtle background noise, such as the sound of a water fountain, wind chimes, or gentle music, can bring tranquility to a space. Consider incorporating soft sounds that soothe, but avoid overly stimulating music or loud noises. If your space has loud outside noises, adding heavy curtains or rugs can help to absorb sound and create a more peaceful atmosphere.

- **Touch**: The textures of your furniture, cushions, and accessories can affect how at ease you feel. Incorporating tactile elements like soft blankets, plush rugs, or smooth wooden surfaces can invite comfort and relaxation. Textures can also be useful in the bedroom or meditation spaces, where comfort and softness are key to relaxation and focus. Consider integrating natural materials like wood, cotton, and linen to create a warm, inviting space.

- **Smell**: The scent of a room can have a profound effect on your mood. Natural scents like lavender, citrus, and sandalwood promote calm and clarity. Scented candles, essential oils, or diffusers can infuse your home with calming aromas. Just remember to keep the scents subtle so that they don't overwhelm the senses. You could also try using herbs like rosemary or fresh flowers to add natural fragrance to your home.

- **Taste**: Taste, though often overlooked in creating a peaceful space, can contribute significantly to the overall ambiance of your home. The act of savoring food or beverages mindfully can be an anchor to the present moment. A piece of dark chocolate, or a bowl of fresh fruit can be more than just sustenance—they can be opportunities for sensory experience. By paying attention to the textures, flavors, and sensations each item offers, you can create small, quiet moments of enjoyment.

Mindful Organization: Creating Zones for Clarity

An organized space isn't just about tidiness; it's about creating zones within your home that foster a sense of purpose and clarity. Each area of your home should have a function that aligns with the atmosphere you want to create. For example, a dedicated reading area should feel quiet and cozy, while a workspace should be conducive to focus and productivity.

When organizing, think about how each area can support the activities you want to engage in. A peaceful space invites you to be present in the moment, so each area should be designed with that intention. Perhaps you'll place your favorite chair by the window for a quiet spot to read, or create a small meditation nook where you can retreat for brief moments of relaxation. Consider the emotional tone of each space and how you want to feel there, whether it's energized, calm, or focused.

Incorporating Nature: Bringing the Outdoors In

Nature has an innate ability to bring calm and tranquility. When possible, introduce natural elements into your home. Plants, flowers, and even natural stone or wood can transform a space into a sanctuary of calm. The presence of plants has been shown to reduce stress and increase productivity, and simply observing the life cycle of a plant—whether it's blooming or shedding leaves—can be a reminder of the natural flow of life.

Small changes like a single plant or a few stones placed thoughtfully around your home can create a connection to nature. Alternatively, you can use images of natural landscapes, or open windows to let in fresh air and natural light. By incorporating nature into your living spaces, you're fostering an environment that invites presence, peace, and grounding.

The Importance of Light and Air

Light plays an essential role in a peaceful space, impacting everything from mood to productivity. Natural light is the most beneficial, so whenever possible, let in sunlight by opening curtains or blinds. The warmth and brightness of natural light can elevate the atmosphere of any room.

If natural light is limited, consider using artificial lighting that mimics daylight. Soft, warm-toned light bulbs can add warmth and reduce harshness. Avoid overly bright lights, which can create a sterile or overstimulating environment. Instead, use lamps or dimmable lights to control the ambiance and create a soothing atmosphere.

Similarly, the air quality in your home is crucial for maintaining a peaceful environment. Open windows regularly to allow fresh air to circulate, and use fans or air purifiers to keep the air clear and pleasant. If you live in a space with limited airflow, indoor plants or essential oil diffusers can improve air quality while also adding a sense of calm to the room.

Creating a Space for Reflection and Growth

Beyond physical elements, creating a peaceful space is about cultivating an environment that fosters inner peace and growth. This might mean dedicating a corner of your home to personal reflection, where you can sit quietly, journal, meditate, or simply be present. A space like this encourages mindfulness and offers a place for you to reconnect with yourself.

In a peaceful space, every item should have a purpose, whether it's a piece of art that brings you joy, a soft pillow that invites you to rest, or a table that holds personal items that bring you comfort. Think of your home as a reflection of your inner self, where the environment nurtures a sense of peace, stillness, and mindfulness.

A Peaceful Space at Home

Creating a peaceful space at home is an intentional process that requires thoughtfulness and care. It's about more than just decluttering or decorating; it's about cultivating an environment that supports your emotional well-being and enhances your ability to be present in the moment. By thoughtfully considering the sensory elements, organization, and atmosphere of your space, you create a sanctuary where mindfulness can thrive.

A peaceful space is a place where you can retreat from the outside world, relax, reflect, and recharge. It's a place where you can engage with yourself fully, whether through rest, work, or creative expression. By dedicating time to craft such an environment, you lay the foundation for a more balanced and mindful life.

CHAPTER 7: THE ROLE OF MINDFULNESS IN FOCUS AND ATTENTION

The Power of Focus and Attention

Focus is an essential skill that shapes our mental clarity and productivity. It is the foundation upon which we build our accomplishments, deepen our relationships, and experience life in its full richness. Our ability to concentrate and stay present with what we are doing is crucial not only for getting tasks done but also for creating meaningful experiences.

The act of focusing isn't just about narrowing our attention —it is about directing our mind with purpose, intention, and presence. It is through the practice of mindfulness that we can strengthen our capacity for focus, overcome distractions, and achieve greater clarity in our daily lives.

In this chapter, we will explore how mindfulness enhances our focus and attention. We will discuss practical techniques that can be applied to train our minds to remain anchored in the present moment, bringing greater depth and clarity to all that we do.

The Role of Focus in Our Daily Lives

Focus plays a central role in every aspect of our lives. It shapes our experiences, influences our ability to learn and retain information, and ultimately determines the quality of our work and relationships.

When we are fully focused, we are fully immersed in the present moment. Our attention is undivided, allowing us to be more productive, creative, and engaged. This sense of engagement enhances the enjoyment of our activities, leading to a deeper satisfaction and sense of accomplishment.

On the other hand, when our focus is scattered or fragmented, we can experience a sense of dissatisfaction and fatigue. We may feel like we are merely going through the motions without truly connecting to the task or the moment. In these instances, mindfulness helps us refocus, bringing our awareness back to what truly matters.

By cultivating mindfulness, we can improve our ability to focus on the present moment and transform our approach to both simple and complex tasks. This practice enables us to be more intentional in how we use our attention and connect with our surroundings.

The Difference Between Shallow and Deep Focus

Focus exists on a spectrum. At one end, we have shallow focus, where our attention is divided, fleeting, or surface-level. Shallow focus occurs when we jump between tasks, mentally multitask, or experience distractions, leading to a feeling of being constantly pulled in different directions. Though we may accomplish tasks during these periods, the quality of our work and the satisfaction we derive from it may be compromised.

On the other end, deep focus represents the highest level of concentration and engagement. It is a state where our attention is fully absorbed by the task at hand. In this state, time seems to fade away, and we are deeply immersed in the process, allowing us to perform at our best. This kind of focus leads to higher quality work, greater creativity, and a deeper sense of satisfaction.

Mindfulness enhances our ability to access and maintain deep focus by training our minds to stay present and avoid distractions. Through regular mindfulness practice, we become more attuned to the present moment and better equipped to sustain attention for longer periods of time.

Techniques for Cultivating Focus with Mindfulness

Mindfulness provides several powerful techniques that can help us train our attention and improve focus. These practices can be incorporated into our daily routines and are designed to increase our ability to concentrate and engage fully with whatever task we are working on.

1. Mindful Breathing

One of the simplest and most effective mindfulness techniques is mindful breathing. By focusing on the breath, we can calm the mind, reduce distractions, and bring ourselves into the present moment. Paying attention to the sensations of breathing helps anchor our attention, providing a foundation for focus.

To practice mindful breathing:

- Sit comfortably in a quiet space.
- Close your eyes and bring your awareness to your breath.
- Notice the sensation of the breath entering and leaving your body.
- If your mind starts to wander, gently guide your attention back to the breath.

Mindful breathing helps you develop the skill of concentrating on one thing at a time, improving your overall ability to focus throughout the day.

2. Single-Tasking with Full Presence

Multitasking is often seen as a skill, but it actually divides our attention and decreases our ability to focus on any one task. Single-tasking, in contrast, involves fully dedicating our attention to one activity at a time. This practice not only improves focus but also enhances the quality of our work.

To practice single-tasking mindfully:

- Choose one task to focus on and eliminate distractions.
- Bring your full attention to the task at hand.
- If your mind starts to wander, gently bring it back to the task.
- Complete the task before moving on to the next one.

Single-tasking allows for deeper engagement and concentration, making it easier to accomplish tasks with greater ease and precision.

3. Mindful Pauses

Mindful pauses are intentional breaks that help refresh the mind and bring back focus. In between tasks or during moments of mental fatigue, taking a mindful pause helps reset the brain, making it easier to return to work with renewed attention.

A mindful pause can be as simple as taking a few deep breaths or stretching. During these brief moments, focus solely on your breath or the sensations in your body.

To practice mindful pauses:

- Set aside moments throughout the day to pause and reset.
- Close your eyes and take a few slow, deep breaths.
- Notice the sensations in your body and bring awareness to the present moment.
- If you have time, stand up and stretch or walk for a few minutes.

Taking regular mindful pauses helps maintain your energy and focus throughout the day.

4. Visualization for Focus

Visualization is a technique used by athletes, artists, and performers to mentally rehearse an activity or goal. By visualizing success, we mentally prepare ourselves to approach a task with focus and clarity.

To practice visualization for focus:

- Find a quiet space and close your eyes.
- Picture yourself successfully completing the task at hand, paying attention to the details of the process.
- Imagine yourself focused, calm, and engaged throughout the task.
- Visualize the satisfaction and sense of accomplishment once the task is completed.

Visualization helps prime the mind for focused action, making it easier to concentrate and complete tasks with intention.

5. The "Stop and Focus" Practice

The "Stop and Focus" practice is a quick mindfulness technique designed to help you return to the present moment when distractions arise. It is especially useful when you find yourself feeling overwhelmed or mentally scattered.

To practice the "Stop and Focus" technique:

- Pause for a moment and take a deep breath.
- Close your eyes or lower your gaze, and bring your attention to your breath.
- Ground yourself in the present moment by noticing the sensations in your body or the environment around you.
- Gently redirect your attention back to the task at hand.

This technique helps you regain focus quickly, allowing you to approach tasks with clarity and intention.

The Path to Enhanced Focus

Focus is a skill that can be cultivated and strengthened with practice. By incorporating mindfulness techniques such as mindful breathing, single-tasking, mindful pauses, visualization, and the "Stop and Focus" practice, you can improve your attention, enhance productivity, and experience greater clarity in everything you do.

Mindfulness helps you train your mind to stay anchored in the present, reducing distractions and fostering deep focus. As you continue to practice mindfulness, you will find that your ability to focus becomes stronger, more effortless, and more rewarding. In turn, this focus will enhance not only your work but also your sense of fulfillment and presence in daily life.

Focus is a cornerstone of success, whether in work, learning, or personal pursuits. It's the ability to direct and maintain attention on a task, ignoring distractions and avoiding mental fatigue. However, in a world that is constantly presenting opportunities for distraction, achieving and sustaining focus can feel increasingly difficult. This is where mindfulness comes into play.

Mindfulness is the practice of staying fully present in the moment—aware of your thoughts, feelings, and surroundings without becoming distracted by what has passed or what is to come. This awareness, when applied to our tasks, can significantly enhance our ability to concentrate, reduce mental clutter, and enable us to direct our energy toward what truly matters. In this chapter, we will explore how mindfulness helps us remain focused, the importance of mindful pauses, and how mindfulness supports us in staying on track despite the natural distractions of our minds.

How Mindfulness Helps Us Stay Present and Maintain Deep Concentration

The human mind is naturally inclined to wander. Thoughts drift from one topic to another, sometimes even unrelated to the task at hand. It might be a fleeting worry about something in the future, a reflection on an experience from the past, or just a random idea that pops up. This wandering is a normal part of the thinking process, but it can undermine our ability to concentrate. The more our minds wander, the harder it becomes to return to the task and maintain deep concentration.

Mindfulness provides a way to navigate this tendency by helping us bring our attention back to the present moment. It encourages us to acknowledge our thoughts without judgment, to notice when our attention has drifted, and to gently guide it back to what we were focusing on. Instead of getting frustrated with ourselves for being distracted, mindfulness offers us the space to recognize the distraction and choose to refocus with intention.

Through regular practice, mindfulness allows us to strengthen our capacity to concentrate. When we cultivate mindfulness, we develop an awareness of where our focus is at any given moment, and we gain the skill to return to the present whenever our minds wander. This skill not only enhances our ability to focus in the moment, but it also builds the foundation for deeper, more sustained concentration.

This deep focus, often referred to as "flow," is a state in which we become fully immersed in an activity. In this state, we lose track of time and experience heightened productivity and creativity. Achieving flow is easier when we practice mindfulness, as it trains the mind to stay present, allowing us to fully engage with the task at hand. Mindfulness supports flow by eliminating the distractions that otherwise prevent us from achieving this heightened state of focus.

The Benefits of Mindful Pauses and Short Breaks

While maintaining focus is important, so too is allowing our minds the opportunity to rest. Many people make the mistake of trying to power through hours of work or study without pausing, but this can lead to mental fatigue and diminished focus. Instead, taking mindful pauses—short breaks to clear your mind and reconnect with the present moment—can significantly enhance concentration.

Mindful pauses don't require much time or effort. These breaks might involve closing your eyes for a few seconds to breathe deeply, feeling the sensations in your body, or simply sitting in stillness for a moment. Such pauses create an opportunity for the mind to reset, reducing stress and fatigue. It's during these brief moments of rest that we can regain mental clarity and energy, returning to our tasks with refreshed focus.

Regular mindful breaks also help prevent burnout. Working without breaks can lead to mental overload, making it harder to concentrate and increasing the likelihood of mistakes. Mindful pauses, on the other hand, help balance the mental exertion required by focused tasks with moments of relaxation, ensuring sustained energy and clarity.

Furthermore, taking breaks allows us to reflect on our progress. During a mindful pause, we might notice that our attention has been divided or that we've drifted from our original intention. These moments of reflection provide an opportunity to re-align with our goals and clarify our next steps. In this way, mindful breaks not only restore our focus but also guide us in making necessary adjustments, keeping us on track and moving forward with purpose.

Using Mindfulness to Combat Distractions

Distractions are a natural part of life, and they aren't always external. Sometimes, the greatest distractions come from within—our wandering thoughts, emotional reactions, or even physical discomfort. Mindfulness provides a powerful tool for addressing these internal distractions. By developing a heightened awareness of what's happening in our minds and bodies, we can learn to recognize when our attention is shifting and intervene before we lose focus entirely.

When we practice mindfulness, we train ourselves to notice

when we're being pulled away from the task at hand. Whether it's a worry about something in the future or a memory from the past, mindfulness teaches us to observe these thoughts without getting entangled in them. We can acknowledge that these thoughts are present but choose not to follow them. Instead of letting them take us away from our focus, we bring our attention back to the task, choosing to remain anchored in the present moment.

This awareness can also help us become more attuned to the physical sensations that often accompany distractions. For example, if you're sitting at a desk and start to feel discomfort in your body—tightness in your back, an aching neck, or a restless feeling in your legs—mindfulness helps you acknowledge these sensations without letting them take over. By paying attention to the sensations and adjusting your posture or taking a brief stretch, you can address the physical distraction before it undermines your focus.

Mindfulness also helps us cultivate patience and self-compassion in the face of distractions. It's easy to become frustrated when we can't maintain concentration, but mindfulness teaches us to observe those frustrations without judgment. We learn that it's natural for the mind to wander, and that the key is not to get frustrated but to return to our focus with gentleness and understanding. This non-judgmental approach reduces the mental resistance that often makes distractions worse, allowing us to refocus with ease.

Mindfulness as a Tool for Improved Focus

Mindfulness is a powerful tool for improving focus. It teaches us to stay present, to recognize when our attention has wandered, and to return to the task at hand with greater intention. By incorporating mindful pauses into our routine, we can prevent mental burnout and ensure that we maintain our energy and clarity throughout the day. And by using mindfulness to address internal and external distractions, we can create a mental environment conducive to deep concentration.

The more we practice mindfulness, the better we become at maintaining focus. This ability to concentrate improves not only our productivity but also our sense of accomplishment and satisfaction. Focus, when cultivated through mindfulness, becomes not just a skill but a way of being—allowing us to fully engage with our work, our relationships, and our lives.

How Mindfulness Helps Us Stay Present and Maintain Deep Concentration

At its simplest, mindfulness is the practice of paying attention, on purpose, in the present moment, and doing so without judgment. When it comes to focus, mindfulness teaches us to fully engage with whatever task we are working on, removing ourselves from the constant internal chatter and the external noise that so often disrupts our concentration.

Our minds have a natural tendency to wander. Our thoughts often drift away from what we should be focusing on. This wandering, known as "mind-wandering," can cause a significant decrease in productivity. The more our attention shifts away from the task at hand, the harder it becomes to return to it. But mindfulness offers a way to retrain this process. By observing our thoughts without judgment, we can gently guide our attention back to the task at hand.

Practicing mindfulness regularly helps us develop a better capacity for attention control. Over time, it teaches us to recognize when our attention has strayed and helps us return to the present moment with intention and clarity. The more we practice staying focused on a single point of attention, the easier it becomes to maintain deep concentration. It's not about forcing ourselves to ignore distractions, but about acknowledging them without becoming entangled in them, and then returning our focus back to what's important. This is a practice, and like any skill, the more we train, the better we become.

Mindfulness can also help us develop what is often called "deep focus" or "flow." In these states, we become fully immersed in the activity we're doing. Time seems to stand still, and we experience a heightened sense of clarity and productivity. Flow states are not only beneficial for getting things done—they also make tasks more enjoyable. And mindfulness is key to entering and maintaining flow. By staying present and engaged with the task at hand, we can increase our chances of entering these focused, productive states where distractions fade away.

Training the Brain for Focus

One of the most powerful effects of mindfulness is its ability to train the brain. Just like any other skill, focus can be developed and improved through consistent practice. When we regularly practice mindfulness, we are strengthening the neural pathways associated with attention and focus. These pathways help us concentrate more effectively, filter out irrelevant stimuli, and return to a state of focus more quickly after we've been distracted.

Mindfulness also enhances cognitive flexibility, the ability to switch focus between different tasks without losing efficiency. Cognitive flexibility is an important skill in today's world, where we often juggle multiple responsibilities and switch between tasks. Mindfulness helps us become more adept at this skill by teaching us to stay grounded in the present moment, regardless of how many things are demanding our attention.

Focus as a Cognitive Skill

Focus, as a cognitive skill, is essential for achieving success in any area of life. It plays a crucial role in productivity, creativity, and even our sense of accomplishment. But focus is also increasingly hard to maintain. Distractions come at us from all angles. In the midst of these interruptions, staying present and concentrated becomes more challenging. This is where mindfulness steps in.

Mindfulness, at its core, is about being fully present in the moment—aware of your thoughts, feelings, and surroundings, without being distracted by what happened earlier or worrying about what might come next. It is this kind of mental presence that can transform your ability to focus. Through mindfulness, you can train your mind to stay anchored in the task at hand, improving your ability to concentrate for longer periods and reducing the effects of distractions. This chapter will explore how mindfulness supports deep concentration, the importance of mindful breaks, and how it can combat the constant distractions of modern life.

CHAPTER 8: MINDFULNESS AND TIME MANAGEMENT

The Relationship Between Mindfulness and Time Management

Effective time management is often perceived as a skill that can be learned through organizing tasks and creating schedules. However, without a deeper understanding of how we approach time, even the most meticulously planned days can feel rushed and out of control. This is where mindfulness plays an essential role. By cultivating mindfulness, we can develop a more aware, intentional relationship with our time. Mindfulness, the practice of being fully present in the moment without judgment, offers the opportunity to reshape how we experience and use time in our daily lives.

Mindfulness teaches us to engage fully with the present moment rather than rushing ahead to the future or dwelling on the past. This practice helps us to notice how we typically use our time, enabling us to make choices that align with our values and priorities. It fosters the ability to focus on one task at a time, reducing distractions and multitasking, which can overwhelm and scatter our attention. This deeper presence allows us to be more intentional in how we allocate time, helping to ensure that our energy is invested in areas that matter most.

One of the first ways mindfulness can support time management is by helping us become more aware of how we spend our time. Often, we go through the motions of the day without truly considering the choices we are making, whether that involves how long we spend on particular tasks or how frequently we allow interruptions to divert our attention. By practicing mindfulness, we can observe how we use our time and, in turn, create more intentional patterns. This awareness acts as the first step toward better time management, as it opens up the possibility for reflection and change.

Mindfulness is particularly effective in reducing the tendency to overcommit ourselves. When we are more mindful of our own energy, we become more adept at setting boundaries and recognizing when we are taking on too much. Mindfulness encourages us to tune into our feelings and body sensations, allowing us to gauge whether we have the capacity for additional tasks. This helps us avoid the burnout that often comes with an overpacked schedule, as mindfulness fosters the ability to assess our limits realistically.

One of the core principles of mindfulness is the ability to focus on the present moment. This principle can be applied to how we manage time by encouraging us to focus on one thing at a time. Multitasking, while often seen as a necessary skill, tends to diminish our overall productivity and increases the cognitive load. When we split our attention between several tasks, each task receives less of our full mental capacity. Mindfulness counteracts this tendency by emphasizing single-tasking, allowing us to direct our full attention to one task and complete it with greater clarity and efficiency. This focused approach to time not only enhances productivity but also allows for a more satisfying and meaningful experience of each task.

Strategies for Mindful Time Management

1. Mindful Awareness of Time

The first step in integrating mindfulness into time management is developing awareness of how we spend our time. Most people operate on autopilot throughout their day, moving from one task to the next without much thought about how much time they are devoting to each activity or whether they are truly focused on the task at hand. Mindfulness encourages us to pause and take stock of our time, observing how we spend it without judgment.

For example, you may find that you spend more time on certain tasks or activities than you realize, or that you're regularly distracted during important tasks. By bringing mindful attention to these moments, you can begin to notice patterns in your time use. You might notice that you often waste time on tasks that aren't aligned with your goals, or that you feel stressed or overwhelmed by a backlog of work. Mindfulness offers a mirror, allowing you to see exactly where your time is going and to identify areas where changes can be made.

2. Mindful Prioritization

Mindfulness also plays a critical role in helping us prioritize our time effectively. Without mindfulness, it's easy to let external demands dictate our schedule, leading to a reactive approach to time management. We end up scrambling to meet deadlines or reacting to interruptions instead of consciously deciding where to invest our time and energy.

By practicing mindfulness, we become more in tune with our values, goals, and true priorities. When we are clear on what truly matters to us, we are better able to make decisions about how to allocate our time. This means we are less likely to spend time on activities that don't align with our long-term objectives or distract us from our core responsibilities.

Mindful prioritization involves regularly checking in with ourselves to assess whether our current tasks align with our most important goals. This process helps us separate the urgent from the important, and it encourages us to be intentional in choosing which tasks deserve our attention. With mindfulness, we can evaluate what will bring us closer to our goals and focus our energy on those activities.

3. Single-Tasking Through Mindfulness

Multitasking is often viewed as a necessary skill, but research has shown that it can lead to decreased efficiency and increased cognitive load. When we attempt to juggle multiple tasks at once, our attention becomes divided, and we become less effective at each task. Mindfulness encourages us to approach tasks one at a time, a practice known as single-tasking.

Single-tasking, with the support of mindfulness, allows us to bring our full attention to one task and fully engage with it. This not only enhances the quality of our work but also helps us experience greater satisfaction from the process. By focusing solely on the task at hand, we are able to work more efficiently, make fewer mistakes, and feel a sense of accomplishment when we complete a task.

The key to single-tasking is to eliminate distractions and direct all our attention to one activity. This can be achieved through mindful breathing or setting clear intentions before starting a task. Mindfulness allows us to notice when our attention is drifting, helping us gently refocus and stay present with the task we are doing.

4. Mindful Decision-Making and Time Allocation

Effective time management is also about making informed decisions about where to spend our time. Often, we may make decisions based on urgency, external pressure, or habit rather than conscious choice. Mindfulness provides the mental space to assess each decision thoughtfully and consider the long-term impact of how we allocate our time.

Before committing to a new task, project, or activity, mindfulness encourages us to pause and ask whether this choice aligns with our priorities and current responsibilities. By practicing mindful decision-making, we avoid the trap of over-scheduling or engaging in tasks that do not support our larger goals. Additionally, mindful time allocation allows us to maintain a balance between work, personal life, and rest, ensuring that we don't neglect important aspects of our lives.

5. Managing Interruptions and Distractions

In the course of our day, interruptions and distractions are inevitable. From phone calls to emails to spontaneous conversations, we are constantly pulled away from our tasks. Mindfulness offers strategies to manage these interruptions more effectively by increasing our awareness of when distractions arise and helping us return to the task at hand.

When faced with an interruption, mindfulness allows us to pause, acknowledge the distraction without judgment, and decide how to respond. We can take a few deep breaths to reset our focus, set boundaries with others, or create environments conducive to fewer distractions. Mindfulness helps us respond to interruptions calmly and with intention, rather than reacting impulsively or allowing the distractions to derail our time management efforts.

6. Reflection and Adjustment

One of the most important aspects of mindfulness in time management is the practice of reflection. Regularly taking time to reflect on how we use our time helps us identify what is working and what needs to be adjusted. Mindfulness encourages us to evaluate our time management strategies without judgment, looking at where we succeeded and where we can improve.

Through regular reflection, we become more adept at identifying areas where we may be wasting time, procrastinating, or allowing distractions to take over. This reflection process allows us to make adjustments, try new strategies, and continually improve our approach to time management. By adopting a mindful approach to reflection, we create a dynamic and flexible time management system that adapts to our needs and priorities.

7. Focusing on the Task at Hand

Mindfulness also helps us manage our time by encouraging us to be present with the task at hand, allowing us to fully engage with what we are doing. When we are focused on the present, we experience a deeper connection to the activity, which often results in greater satisfaction and improved performance. This sense of presence transforms routine activities into meaningful experiences, helping us to find fulfillment and purpose even in the smallest tasks. As we embrace mindfulness, we learn to slow down, savoring the quality of our engagement rather than rushing to the next task or outcome.

8. Mindful Prioritization

Another key aspect of mindful time management is the ability to prioritize. Often, we are overwhelmed with tasks that seem equally urgent, leading to a sense of paralysis or confusion. Mindfulness invites us to approach these decisions with clarity, allowing us to assess which tasks align most with our values and goals. By practicing mindfulness, we are better able to sort through competing demands on our time and make intentional choices about what deserves our attention. This process of prioritization ensures that we are not just reacting to the pressures of the moment but actively choosing how we want to invest our time.

In addition to helping us prioritize, mindfulness can also improve our decision-making. Instead of rushing through decisions or reacting impulsively, mindfulness gives us the space to reflect, consider our options, and respond thoughtfully. When we take a mindful approach to decision-making, we are less likely to fall into the trap of making hasty or emotional choices. We can approach time management with a sense of calm and clear-headedness, ensuring that each decision we make aligns with our broader intentions.

The Role of Mindfulness in Time Management

Mindfulness also enhances time management by helping us resist the impulse to engage in time-wasting activities. In moments of stress or pressure, we may be more likely to procrastinate or turn to distractions for relief. Mindfulness helps us recognize these tendencies as they arise, allowing us to make more conscious choices about how we spend our time. Rather than falling into old habits, we can choose to redirect our energy toward tasks that move us closer to our goals.

The role of mindfulness in time management extends beyond our work-related tasks. It can also support our personal life, helping us find a balance between work, rest, and recreation. By approaching time management mindfully, we can ensure that we are taking the time to care for our physical and mental health. Rather than overcommitting to work or other obligations, mindfulness encourages us to schedule time for self-care, relaxation, and connection with others. This holistic approach to time management ensures that we are not only productive but also well-rested, emotionally balanced, and connected to our own well-being.

At the heart of mindful time management is the practice of being present. By developing the ability to focus on the here and now, we free ourselves from the distractions of worry and anxiety about the future or regrets about the past. Instead of feeling overwhelmed by the tasks ahead, we can approach each moment with calmness and clarity. By living in the present, we become more attuned to how we are using our time and make choices that reflect our true priorities. As a result, we create more space for the things that matter most, whether that is our work, relationships, or personal growth.

Ultimately, mindfulness helps us live in alignment with our values. It allows us to step back from the hustle and bustle of life and reflect on what truly matters. Instead of getting caught up in external pressures or distractions, we can focus on what brings us joy, fulfillment, and purpose. By incorporating mindfulness into our time management practices, we can create a life that feels intentional, balanced, and meaningful. Through this mindful approach to time, we are empowered to make the most of each day, creating the space and clarity needed to live with greater purpose and satisfaction.

In conclusion, mindfulness offers a powerful tool for improving time management. By cultivating mindfulness, we become more aware of how we spend our time, better equipped to prioritize tasks, and more focused on the present moment. Mindful pauses and intentional choices help us resist distractions and overcome procrastination, while also ensuring that we make time for the things that matter most. Through mindfulness, we can approach time management with greater clarity, balance, and purpose, leading to a more fulfilling and productive life.

CHAPTER 9: MINDFUL LISTENING AND COMMUNICATION CULTIVATING DEEPER CONNECTIONS THROUGH AWARENESS

Communication is an essential part of our lives, influencing every relationship we have—whether personal or professional. The way we engage in conversation can either build bridges or create barriers between us. Often, our communication is rushed, distracted, or surface-level, which prevents us from truly connecting with others. Mindful listening, on the other hand, brings us into a deeper, more authentic engagement with the people around us, allowing for better understanding, compassion, and connection. In this chapter, we explore how cultivating mindfulness in our listening can transform the way we communicate, fostering deeper connections in all aspects of our lives.

The Power of Being Present

At the core of mindful listening is being fully present in

the moment. Often, when we listen to others, our minds are occupied with thoughts about what we want to say next, judgments about what is being said, or distractions from the environment around us. In these moments, we may think we are hearing the person, but in reality, we are not fully engaging. True listening requires giving someone our undivided attention. It means not just hearing the words, but also understanding the emotions, intentions, and energy behind them.

Being present in a conversation allows you to absorb what the other person is truly saying. It can help you pick up on subtle nuances—the tone of their voice, their body language, the pause between words, and the emotions that lie beneath the surface. When you are not focused on your own thoughts, you become attuned to the other person's experience, creating a space for true connection and empathy.

To practice being present while listening, start by focusing on your breath. Gently bring your awareness to each inhale and exhale, allowing your body to relax and settle into the moment. When your mind begins to wander or you feel distracted, gently redirect your attention back to the person speaking. This simple act of grounding yourself through breath can be transformative in creating an open, mindful space for communication.

Listening Without Judgment

Another key element of mindful listening is letting go of judgment. When we listen through the lens of judgment, we may be quick to form opinions or jump to conclusions before the other person has finished speaking. We might judge their ideas, tone, or even the way they express themselves. But judgment limits our ability to truly hear and understand them. It also fosters an environment of defensiveness, where both parties feel the need to protect their own perspectives instead of sharing openly.

Mindful listening, in contrast, is about creating a space where we suspend judgment. It means allowing the person to speak freely without feeling the need to analyze, critique, or solve their problems immediately. Instead, we listen with the intention of understanding them on a deeper level, which opens up possibilities for better communication and genuine connection.

By practicing mindfulness in our conversations, we can cultivate an attitude of openness, curiosity, and acceptance. This not only helps us better understand others but also fosters a more supportive and empathetic environment for communication.

Fostering Emotional Awareness

Mindful listening is not only about hearing words but also about recognizing the emotions that accompany them. When we listen mindfully, we are tuned in to the emotions that underlie the conversation. This level of emotional awareness can deepen our connections with others, as it shows that we care not only about what they are saying but also about how they feel.

In a conversation, it is essential to listen to both the content and the emotional tone. Often, the most important parts of a conversation are not explicitly stated. For example, a person may say they are "fine," but their tone, body language, or facial expressions may indicate otherwise. By paying close attention to these subtleties, we can offer more compassionate responses and respond more appropriately to the person's needs.

When we approach conversations with an open heart, we create a space for emotional safety. The person speaking feels heard and understood, and we, in turn, gain a richer understanding of their emotional experience. This deeper level of empathy helps to strengthen relationships and build trust over time.

Mindful Communication in Practice

The practice of mindful listening extends beyond simply being present or suspending judgment; it involves actively engaging in the conversation in a way that fosters mutual respect, clarity, and understanding. Mindful communication is not just about listening to the words but also about ensuring that our own communication is intentional, clear, and respectful.

One way to incorporate mindful communication is through the practice of pausing. When the other person finishes speaking, take a moment to absorb what they have said before responding. This pause creates space for reflection and prevents knee-jerk reactions. It also ensures that your response is thoughtful and aligns with the conversation's tone.

Another useful practice is to reflect back or paraphrase what the other person has said. This not only confirms that you are listening but also helps clarify any misunderstandings. For example, you might say, "What I'm hearing is that you feel frustrated because..." This shows that you are actively listening and striving to understand their perspective.

Silence as a Powerful Tool

In any conversation, silence can be as powerful as words. Mindful listening often involves allowing silence to exist within the conversation. The act of holding space for silence can create a deeper connection and provide an opportunity for both parties to process and reflect. It can also encourage more thoughtful and measured responses.

Silence does not have to be uncomfortable. In fact, it can be quite profound. Pausing after someone speaks gives them room to expand on their thoughts or allows both parties to reflect on what has been shared. Silence invites contemplation, understanding, and connection without the need to fill the space with words.

The Impact of Mindful Listening on Relationships

In both personal and professional settings, mindful listening fosters a sense of respect, trust, and connection. When we listen mindfully, we show the other person that we value their thoughts, feelings, and experiences. This leads to better communication, fewer misunderstandings, and more meaningful relationships.

In personal relationships, mindful listening encourages intimacy and emotional support. It allows partners, friends, and family members to feel safe and understood. It also enables us to respond more effectively to the needs of others, leading to more fulfilling and harmonious interactions.

In the workplace, mindful listening can improve teamwork, collaboration, and leadership. By practicing mindful listening, we become better communicators and problem-solvers. We are more open to others' ideas and more able to contribute meaningfully to group discussions. Mindful listening helps reduce conflict and fosters a culture of respect and understanding, ultimately improving workplace dynamics and productivity.

Listening as an Act of Service

Mindful listening can also be seen as an act of service. When we take the time to truly listen to someone, we are offering them the gift of our full attention and presence. This can be especially important when the other person is going through a difficult time or has important feelings to express. In these moments, our mindful listening can provide comfort, clarity, and support, strengthening the bond between us and the person speaking.

Listening with mindfulness can create a deeper connection to those we care about, showing that we are not merely hearing their words, but fully engaging with their experiences. It is a simple yet powerful way to show empathy, care, and love.

Mindful Listening as a Skill

Mindful listening is an essential skill that can transform our relationships and deepen our connections with others. By cultivating the ability to be present, suspend judgment, and engage with empathy and emotional awareness, we can improve our communication and foster a more meaningful, compassionate way of relating to others. Whether in personal relationships or professional settings, mindful listening helps create an environment of trust, respect, and understanding. It is a simple yet profound practice that, when applied consistently, can enrich our interactions and strengthen our bonds with the people around us. By listening mindfully, we not only enhance our communication but also nurture the connections that bring depth and fulfillment to our lives.

CHAPTER 10: OVERCOMING MENTAL BLOCKS AND PROCRASTINATION

Mental blocks and procrastination are two of the most common barriers to success. They arise when the mind resists engaging with tasks, often without any clear reason. This resistance can feel like a heavy weight, preventing progress and delaying the completion of important work. Overcoming these mental obstacles is not only essential for productivity but also for personal growth and development.

In this chapter, we will explore how mental blocks and procrastination manifest, the underlying causes of these behaviors, and most importantly, how to overcome them. By understanding the psychological mechanisms at play and employing effective strategies, we can break free from these patterns and foster a mindset of proactive engagement and sustained focus.

1. Understanding Mental Blocks

Mental blocks are periods of mental stagnation, where the mind feels stuck and unable to make progress. These blocks can occur in various situations, such as when we are trying to complete a task, make decisions, or find creative solutions. During a mental block, the mind seems to be incapable of generating ideas or making decisions.

These blocks can be frustrating because they often appear without warning. We might sit down to work on something, only to find that our minds are clouded, unable to focus, or paralyzed by uncertainty. In some cases, we may feel an overwhelming sense of frustration or anxiety, which further compounds the block.

The causes of mental blocks can vary from person to person. Often, they are linked to feelings of fear, doubt, or pressure. For instance, fear of failure or a lack of self-confidence can create mental resistance to tackling a task. Similarly, perfectionism, the desire to complete a task perfectly, can prevent us from even starting. Mental blocks are a natural part of the human experience, but they do not need to control us.

2. The Psychology of Procrastination

Procrastination is the act of delaying or postponing tasks, often in favor of less important or more enjoyable activities. While procrastination is often associated with laziness, it is much more complex than that. It is a psychological phenomenon that involves avoiding a task, even when we know that completing it would be beneficial.

At its core, procrastination is rooted in our desire to avoid discomfort. We may procrastinate because we associate a task with negative emotions, such as stress, anxiety, or boredom. This avoidance is an attempt to reduce the emotional discomfort associated with the task at hand. Ironically, procrastination often leads to increased stress, guilt, and anxiety as deadlines approach, creating a vicious cycle of avoidance.

Procrastination can also be driven by a lack of motivation, poor time management skills, or an inability to prioritize tasks. In some cases, individuals procrastinate because they are overwhelmed by the scope of the task or are unsure where to begin. This hesitation can be exacerbated by a lack of clear goals or a sense of uncertainty about the desired outcome.

Understanding the root causes of procrastination is essential for overcoming it. By recognizing the emotional and psychological triggers behind procrastination, we can take proactive steps to break the cycle and build a more productive mindset.

3. Breaking Through Mental Blocks

One of the first steps in overcoming a mental block is to recognize that it is a temporary condition. Mental blocks are not permanent, and they do not define our ability to accomplish tasks. Once we accept that the block is a natural part of the creative or working process, we can begin to address it with the right strategies.

One effective method for overcoming mental blocks is to simply take a break. Sometimes, stepping away from the task at hand allows the mind to reset and gain a fresh perspective. During this break, engage in an activity that allows your mind to relax and unwind. This could be something physical, such as taking a walk, or something creative, like sketching or journaling. The goal is to distract the mind long enough to release the tension that is contributing to the block.

Another approach is to break the task down into smaller, more manageable parts. Large tasks can often feel overwhelming, leading to mental paralysis. When faced with a daunting project, try to divide it into smaller steps or stages. Focusing on completing one small part at a time reduces the pressure and makes the task feel less insurmountable. By concentrating on one step at a time, we can gradually build momentum and overcome the mental block.

Additionally, changing your environment can help reset your mental state. If you have been working in the same space for a long time, it can help to shift your surroundings. A new setting can refresh your mind and provide the mental space needed to overcome the block. This change can be as simple as rearranging your workspace or moving to a different room. Sometimes, even small changes in our environment can provide the mental shift needed to regain focus and clarity.

4. Tackling Procrastination: Strategies for Action

Procrastination can be particularly challenging because it often involves avoiding the very tasks that would move us closer to our goals. The key to overcoming procrastination lies in shifting our mindset and creating actionable steps that make starting and completing tasks easier.

One effective strategy for overcoming procrastination is the use of time-blocking. Time-blocking involves setting aside specific blocks of time to work on a particular task or project. By allocating focused time to a task, you create a sense of urgency and reduce the likelihood of putting it off. This technique helps to eliminate distractions and keeps the mind focused on the task at hand.

A related strategy is the Pomodoro technique, which involves working for 25 minutes followed by a 5-minute break. This method helps combat procrastination by creating a structure that limits the amount of time spent on any one task, making it feel less daunting. By breaking tasks into short, focused intervals, the mind is less likely to resist starting or continuing the work.

Another strategy to combat procrastination is to focus on the "why" behind the task. Reminding yourself of the reasons you want to complete a task can provide the motivation needed to get started. Instead of focusing on how difficult or unpleasant the task may seem, try to concentrate on the positive outcomes that will result from completing it. Whether it's a sense of accomplishment, relief, or the satisfaction of moving closer to your goals, focusing on the benefits can provide the mental push necessary to overcome procrastination.

Additionally, it is important to recognize that perfectionism is often a driving force behind procrastination. Many people procrastinate because they fear that their work will not meet their own high standards. In these cases, it can be helpful to adjust your mindset by setting realistic expectations. Recognize that no task will be perfect, and that starting and making progress is far more important than achieving perfection. By shifting your focus from perfection to progress, you can break free from the paralysis that perfectionism creates.

5. Building Self-Discipline and Motivation

Both mental blocks and procrastination are closely tied to our ability to self-regulate and manage our motivation. Building self-discipline is an essential part of overcoming these obstacles. Self-discipline is the ability to control our impulses, focus on long-term goals, and make consistent progress, even when it feels difficult.

One way to build self-discipline is to establish clear goals and create a plan of action. When we have a roadmap for what we want to achieve, it becomes easier to stay on track. Break your goals down into smaller, actionable steps and make sure each step is measurable and achievable. By setting clear intentions and tracking progress, you create a sense of accountability and purpose that drives motivation.

Additionally, creating a consistent routine can help build the habit of focusing on important tasks. When we follow a regular schedule, our bodies and minds begin to associate specific activities with certain times of the day, reducing the likelihood of procrastination. Routines create structure and ensure that we allocate time for important tasks, even when motivation is lacking.

Accountability can also play a significant role in overcoming procrastination. By sharing your goals with others, whether it's a friend, colleague, or mentor, you create external pressure to stay on task. Knowing that someone else is aware of your commitments can encourage you to follow through and prevent delays.

6. Embracing Imperfection and Progress

Finally, it's important to embrace imperfection and recognize that progress is more important than perfection. Many people procrastinate because they are overwhelmed by the desire to do everything perfectly. Perfectionism can be paralyzing and prevent us from making any progress at all. Instead, focus on taking small steps forward and making progress, even if it's not flawless.

By embracing imperfection, we free ourselves from the fear of failure and the belief that we must do everything flawlessly. Every step forward, no matter how small, brings us closer to our goals. The key is to remain consistent and focused on the process, rather than obsessing over the end result.

Overcoming Mental Blocks

Mental blocks and procrastination are natural challenges that everyone faces at some point. However, they do not need to control our actions or outcomes. By recognizing the underlying causes of mental resistance, we can employ strategies to overcome these obstacles and regain focus. Whether it's by breaking tasks into smaller steps, using time-blocking techniques, adjusting our mindset, or building self-discipline, there are countless ways to manage procrastination and break through mental blocks.

Ultimately, overcoming mental blocks and procrastination requires patience, persistence, and a willingness to take action. By building consistent habits and adopting a mindset that values progress over perfection, we can break free from these barriers and unlock our full potential.

CHAPTER 11: THE POWER OF REST AND RECOVERY IN ENHANCING PRODUCTIVITY

In the pursuit of high performance and productivity, the importance of rest and recovery is often overlooked. Many individuals believe that the more hours they put into work or study, the more they will achieve. However, the reality is that rest plays an equally crucial role in maintaining focus and sustaining long-term success. This chapter explores the relationship between rest, recovery, and focus, providing insight into how strategic rest can optimize productivity and mental clarity.

1. The Necessity of Rest

Rest plays an essential role in the cognitive processes that supports optimal function. Our brains and bodies are not designed to operate at peak performance without pauses. When we are engaged in focused tasks, whether mentally or physically demanding, our resources are gradually depleted. Without adequate recovery, these resources become exhausted, leading to diminished focus, increased mental fatigue, and reduced efficiency.

Taking deliberate breaks and ensuring proper rest cycles allows us to recharge. This replenishment is necessary for sustaining the energy required for sustained attention, critical thinking, and creative problem-solving. Rest is not a luxury, but a fundamental requirement for maintaining the high level of performance necessary for consistent focus and effective work.

2. The Effect of Mental Fatigue

Mental fatigue is the result of prolonged concentration and mental effort. Just as physical exertion leads to tired muscles, intense mental activity can lead to cognitive exhaustion. When the brain is engaged in demanding tasks, it uses up glucose and other resources, leaving it less capable of sustaining focus and clear thinking over time.

Mental fatigue impacts various cognitive functions, including memory, decision-making, and reaction time. When mental fatigue sets in, individuals often find it difficult to concentrate, think critically, or process information efficiently. This decline in cognitive performance not only affects productivity but can also lead to poor judgment and increased stress levels.

It is at this point that rest becomes crucial. Just as muscles need recovery after intense physical activity, the brain requires rest periods to restore its energy levels and cognitive capacity. In fact, taking regular breaks can prevent cognitive overload, which is a state where the brain becomes so overwhelmed with information that it cannot process it effectively. Regular rest helps reset the brain, allowing it to return to a state of clarity and sharpness.

3. The Importance of Sleep

Sleep is one of the most vital forms of rest for the brain. During sleep, the body and brain undergo a restorative process that is critical for both physical and mental health. While we sleep, our brains consolidate memories, process emotions, and clear out toxins that accumulate during waking hours. These processes are essential for maintaining cognitive function and mental clarity during the day.

The quality of sleep can significantly impact focus and concentration. Adequate, uninterrupted sleep allows the brain to rest and recover fully, ensuring that we wake up refreshed and ready to engage in focused tasks. On the other hand, poor sleep quality or insufficient sleep can impair attention, memory, and decision-making skills. Sleep deprivation can lead to difficulties in maintaining focus and significantly reduce our cognitive abilities.

Developing healthy sleep habits is essential for optimal performance. This includes maintaining a consistent sleep schedule, ensuring that the sleep environment is conducive to rest, and avoiding disruptions before bedtime. When sleep is prioritized as a form of recovery, individuals experience enhanced mental clarity and focus throughout the day.

4. The Role of Rest in Preventing Burnout

Chronic stress and continuous work without adequate recovery often lead to burnout. Burnout is a state of physical, emotional, and mental exhaustion caused by prolonged stress. It can lead to a significant decline in productivity, motivation, and overall well-being. One of the key contributing factors to burnout is the failure to take regular breaks and prioritize recovery.

Rest plays a pivotal role in preventing burnout. By incorporating regular periods of rest into daily routines, individuals can avoid the buildup of stress that contributes to burnout. These breaks allow for mental and emotional rejuvenation, reducing the negative impact of stress. Whether through sleep, relaxation, or simply taking time to pause throughout the day, rest is a protective measure that shields the mind from the long-term effects of stress.

Strategically incorporating rest into your routine is a key preventative measure against burnout. Rather than pushing through fatigue, taking time for rest can help you return to tasks with a renewed sense of energy and focus. This proactive approach to rest ensures that your productivity remains sustainable over time.

5. Active Rest and Its Impact on Focus

While passive rest, such as sleep, is essential, active rest can also be highly beneficial for maintaining focus. Active rest involves engaging in light, restorative activities that promote physical and mental relaxation without demanding the same level of energy or effort as work or strenuous exercise. Activities such as stretching, walking, or deep breathing exercises are examples of active rest that can help reset the mind and body during periods of intense focus.

Active rest helps improve blood circulation, reduce muscle tension, and alleviate mental stress. These activities provide an opportunity for the mind to disengage from the task at hand, preventing cognitive overload and promoting clarity. Active rest also helps maintain a sense of balance throughout the day, ensuring that individuals do not feel mentally or physically drained by prolonged periods of intense focus.

Incorporating active rest into your routine is a simple yet effective strategy for enhancing focus and productivity. By taking short, mindful breaks that engage the body and mind in restorative activities, you can maintain sustained concentration without succumbing to fatigue.

6. Strategic Breaks and Focused Work Sessions

Taking breaks is not just about resting; it is also about timing and structure. The strategic use of breaks can greatly enhance focus and productivity. By organizing your work into focused blocks of time, followed by intentional breaks, you can sustain concentration and avoid burnout. This approach aligns with the body's natural rhythms and ensures that mental energy is used efficiently.

One effective strategy is to divide work into intervals, such as working for 25 to 45 minutes followed by a short break. During these focused work sessions, the mind remains fully engaged, while the breaks allow it to recharge and reset. During breaks, it is important to disengage completely from the task at hand. This mental separation allows the brain to rest and refresh, making it easier to return to the task with renewed energy and focus.

The key to successful breaks is to ensure that they are regular and deliberate. Rather than waiting until you feel mentally drained, taking proactive breaks can help prevent fatigue from setting in. These planned intervals of rest help maintain high levels of focus and reduce the likelihood of mental burnout.

7. The Relationship Between Recovery and Long-Term Focus

Rest and recovery are essential not only for immediate focus but also for long-term cognitive function. Continuous periods of work without rest can lead to diminishing returns, where the quality of work and focus decline over time. In contrast, regular periods of rest, both short-term (such as breaks during the day) and long-term (such as sleep), allow the mind and body to recharge and maintain high levels of performance.

In the long run, the cumulative effects of proper rest and recovery can lead to improved cognitive abilities, sharper focus, and enhanced productivity. By integrating rest into your daily routine and respecting the need for recovery, you set the foundation for sustained focus over the long term. This not only improves your performance in individual tasks but also supports consistent progress toward your broader goals.

8. Rest as a Tool for Mental Clarity

Mental clarity is a key component of focus. When we are well-rested, our minds are clear, organized, and able to process information more effectively. Rest plays a significant role in maintaining mental clarity by allowing the brain to organize thoughts, eliminate distractions, and process information in a more efficient manner.

Taking breaks and getting adequate sleep help clear mental

fog, making it easier to focus on the task at hand. When we are fatigued, our ability to concentrate diminishes, and our thoughts become scattered. Rest helps restore order to the mind, enabling us to approach tasks with greater mental clarity and purpose.

Incorporating rest into your routine is a powerful strategy for enhancing mental clarity and maintaining focus. By prioritizing rest, you create the conditions for clearer thinking, improved decision-making, and a sharper ability to concentrate.

9. Rest as a Component of Self-Care

Rest is an integral aspect of self-care. Just as we care for our physical health through exercise and nutrition, we must also care for our mental health through rest and recovery. Taking the time to rest is an act of self-respect and self-care, ensuring that we can function at our best and remain focused on our goals.

Recognizing the importance of rest is a step toward taking better care of yourself. When rest becomes a regular part of your routine, it shows that you value your well-being and are committed to maintaining a healthy balance between effort and recovery. This balanced approach fosters a sustainable path toward success, where focus and productivity are consistently maintained over time.

Sustaining Focus and Productivity

Rest and recovery are integral to sustaining focus and productivity. Mental fatigue, burnout, and reduced cognitive performance are common consequences of neglecting the need for rest. By prioritizing rest, we ensure that our minds and bodies remain in optimal condition for the tasks at hand. Rest is not a passive activity; it is an active strategy for maintaining mental clarity, preventing burnout, and enhancing focus. Through intentional breaks, proper sleep, and active rest, we can cultivate a sustained, high level of focus and achieve long-term success.

CHAPTER 12: CULTIVATING A POSITIVE MINDSET

A positive mindset is one of the most influential factors in determining how well we can focus on the tasks at hand. The way we perceive and approach challenges significantly impacts our mental state and our ability to maintain attention and clarity. Developing and nurturing a positive mindset is not just about feeling good—it's about training the mind to stay resilient, engaged, and committed, even when faced with distractions or setbacks. In this chapter, we explore how cultivating a positive mindset can enhance focus, and offer practical strategies for developing and maintaining a mindset that fosters productivity, perseverance, and mental clarity.

1. The Connection Between Mindset and Focus

Mindset influences nearly every aspect of our cognitive functioning. A positive mindset primes the brain for greater resilience, better problem-solving, and improved focus. When we approach challenges with optimism and confidence, we create a mental environment that supports sustained attention. In contrast, a negative or fixed mindset can lead to frustration, distraction, and reduced cognitive resources.

A positive mindset helps maintain motivation and energy, especially when tasks become difficult or monotonous. It encourages individuals to stay engaged, even when the task requires long hours of focused effort. By cultivating a mindset that embraces challenge, learning, and growth, we can strengthen our ability to concentrate and direct our mental energy effectively.

2. Overcoming Negative Thought Patterns

Negative thinking can often lead to distractions and impede our ability to focus. When we allow self-doubt, fear, or pessimism to take hold, it becomes difficult to stay present in the task at hand. Such thoughts can create mental clutter, making it harder to direct attention and sustain concentration. Over time, if negative thought patterns are left unchecked, they can diminish both motivation and mental clarity.

To combat negative thought patterns, it can be helpful to practice cognitive restructuring. This involves recognizing negative thoughts as they arise and intentionally shifting them toward more constructive, solution-oriented thinking. By replacing self-critical or discouraging thoughts with positive affirmations, individuals can create a mindset that supports focus and productivity. It is important to understand that negative thoughts are not inherently harmful, but it is our response to them that determines their impact on focus. By reframing challenges as opportunities for growth, the brain becomes more adaptable and resilient.

3. The Power of Self-Compassion

One of the most effective ways to cultivate a positive mindset is through self-compassion. Self-compassion involves treating oneself with the same kindness and understanding that one would offer to a friend. Instead of berating ourselves for mistakes or setbacks, we acknowledge them as part of the human experience and respond with empathy and patience.

When individuals practice self-compassion, they are less likely to become discouraged by failure or frustration. Instead of getting lost in negative emotions, they can refocus their energy on the task at hand. This allows for greater mental flexibility and the ability to bounce back from setbacks without losing momentum. A compassionate mindset makes it easier to stay focused because it removes the emotional baggage that can cloud judgment and divert attention.

Additionally, self-compassion encourages a growth mindset, where individuals view challenges as opportunities for development rather than threats. This shift in perspective makes it easier to stay motivated and focused, even when progress is slow or difficult.

4. Fostering a Growth Mindset

A growth mindset is one in which individuals believe that their abilities and intelligence can be developed over time with effort, learning, and perseverance. This mindset stands in contrast to a fixed mindset, where individuals believe their abilities are static and cannot be changed. When individuals cultivate a growth mindset, they are more likely to embrace challenges, persist in the face of obstacles, and maintain focus on their goals.

The growth mindset also allows individuals to view setbacks as learning opportunities rather than as failures. When faced with difficulty, those with a growth mindset will tend to remain engaged in the process, using the experience as a chance to improve. This perspective is crucial for maintaining focus because it reduces the fear of failure that often causes people to disengage when things become tough.

To foster a growth mindset, individuals should focus on the process rather than the outcome. Celebrating effort, progress, and small victories can reinforce the belief that success is attainable through hard work and perseverance. Additionally, it is important to embrace challenges as part of the journey toward mastery. The more individuals practice a growth mindset, the more it becomes ingrained, creating an environment in which focus and perseverance thrive.

5. The Impact of Positive Self-Talk

Self-talk is the internal dialogue we have with ourselves

throughout the day. It plays a crucial role in shaping our mindset and, by extension, our ability to focus. Positive self-talk helps reinforce a growth mindset, boosts confidence, and supports resilience. When individuals engage in positive self-talk, they are more likely to remain motivated and focused, even in the face of adversity.

Conversely, negative self-talk can undermine focus and create distractions. Phrases like "I can't do this" or "This is too hard" can weaken resolve and make it difficult to stay on track. Over time, negative self-talk can erode confidence and lead to procrastination, mental fatigue, and diminished focus.

To develop a more positive and supportive internal dialogue, we can practice affirmations such as "I can do hard things" and conscious reframing. Instead of focusing on limitations, we can remind ourselves of our strengths, past successes, and potential for growth. By replacing negative thoughts with empowering, encouraging statements, we can enhance this positive mindset and, in turn, our ability to focus.

6. Building Resilience Through Positive Mindset

A positive mindset is not just about feeling good—it can also be about building resilience. Resilience is the ability to recover quickly from setbacks and continue pursuing one's goals, despite challenges. When individuals cultivate a positive mindset, they strengthen their resilience by learning to view obstacles as temporary and manageable. This makes it easier to stay focused and maintain momentum, even when faced with difficulties.

Resilience is essential for focus because it enables individuals to stay engaged in the task at hand, even when things don't go according to plan. Without resilience, setbacks can lead to frustration, loss of motivation, and mental fatigue. However, with a positive mindset that emphasizes perseverance and adaptability, individuals are more likely to bounce back and refocus their attention.

One of the key strategies for building resilience is to focus on what is within one's control. Instead of fixating on external factors that cannot be changed, individuals with a resilient mindset direct their energy toward taking actionable steps that move them closer to their goals. This proactive approach fosters a sense of empowerment, which enhances focus and motivation.

7. Cultivating Mental Flexibility

Mental flexibility is another crucial aspect of a positive mindset. It involves the ability to adapt to changing circumstances and adjust one's thinking in response to new information or challenges. A flexible mind is more capable of maintaining focus because it can easily shift gears when necessary, without becoming stuck in rigid patterns of thought.

Mental flexibility allows individuals to approach tasks with an open mind, which is particularly useful when faced with obstacles or unexpected changes. Those who cultivate mental flexibility are more likely to stay engaged with their work, rather than becoming frustrated or distracted when things don't go as planned.

To develop mental flexibility, individuals can practice embracing uncertainty and reframing challenges as opportunities for learning. They can also cultivate curiosity, remaining open to new ideas and perspectives. The more adaptable one's thinking, the easier it is to stay focused, regardless of the situation.

8. The Role of Visualization in Enhancing Focus

Visualization is a powerful mental technique that can help strengthen focus and build a positive mindset. By imagining success, individuals create a mental blueprint of their goals and the steps required to achieve them. This not only boosts motivation but also helps to clarify the path forward, making it easier to concentrate on the task at hand.

Visualization works by reinforcing the belief that success is attainable, which in turn fosters a mindset that is focused and goal-oriented. By regularly practicing visualization, individuals can program their minds for success, making it easier to stay on task and maintain concentration.

In addition to visualizing success, individuals can also visualize the process of overcoming challenges. This mental rehearsal helps build confidence and resilience, ensuring that individuals are prepared to stay focused, even when obstacles arise.

9. The Role of Emotional Regulation in Focus

Emotional regulation is an essential component of a positive mindset that directly supports our ability to maintain focus. The emotions we experience throughout the day can either enhance or undermine our concentration. For example, intense emotions like frustration, anger, or anxiety can create mental distractions that make it difficult to stay on task, while positive emotions like contentment and motivation can sharpen attention and improve mental clarity. Learning to manage and regulate emotions is therefore crucial for cultivating a mindset that sustains focus.

At its core, emotional regulation involves the ability to recognize, understand, and manage our emotional responses in a way that supports our goals and overall well-being. When we are emotionally overwhelmed or reactive, it can be challenging to concentrate on tasks, as our minds are preoccupied with the emotional experience. In contrast, when we regulate our emotions effectively, we can maintain a calm and focused mental state, even in the face of stress or adversity.

A key aspect of emotional regulation is recognizing the impact emotions have on our cognitive functioning. Strong emotions can trigger a "fight or flight" response, which is hardwired to prioritize immediate action over sustained thought. While this response can be helpful in certain situations, it can hinder focus in others, particularly when complex or sustained attention is required. By learning how to recognize when emotions are becoming overwhelming and taking steps to calm the mind, we can minimize emotional interference and improve our ability to concentrate.

Developing emotional regulation requires a combination of self-awareness and practical strategies. One common approach is mindfulness, which involves paying close attention to one's emotional states without judgment. By practicing mindfulness, individuals can become more attuned to their emotions, allowing them to manage their responses more effectively. Mindfulness techniques such as deep breathing, body scans, or simply pausing to observe emotions as they arise can help individuals detach from intense feelings and return to a place of calm focus.

10. Reframing

Another essential strategy for emotional regulation is reframing. This involves changing the way we think about challenging situations or emotions. For instance, if we encounter an obstacle that causes frustration, we can reframe the situation as an opportunity to learn and grow, rather than as an insurmountable challenge. By shifting our perspective, we reduce the emotional charge attached to the situation, allowing us to stay focused on the task rather than becoming derailed by negative emotions.

Additionally, managing our emotional energy involves setting boundaries and knowing when to take breaks. Overexposure to stressful or emotionally draining situations can deplete our mental energy, making it harder to concentrate. Taking regular breaks to rest and recharge helps to maintain emotional equilibrium, ensuring that we approach tasks with a balanced and focused mindset.

Overall, emotional regulation is an essential skill for sustaining focus over time. By learning how to manage emotions effectively, we can create a mental environment that fosters concentration and mental clarity.

Consistency is Key

While cultivating a positive mindset is a powerful tool for enhancing focus, it requires consistency. A positive mindset is not a one-time effort, but rather a habit that must be nurtured over time. By consistently practicing positive thinking, self-compassion, and resilience, individuals can strengthen their mindset and create an environment in which focus can thrive.

Developing a positive mindset involves regular self-reflection, intentional practice, and a commitment to growth. The more consistently individuals engage in these practices, the more ingrained their positive mindset becomes, resulting in sustained focus and improved performance.

CHAPTER 13: KEEPING A MINDFUL PRESENCE THROUGHOUT THE DAY

Mindfulness is often thought of as something practiced in specific moments: during meditation, on a quiet walk, or during moments of reflection. However, mindfulness, at its core, is about being fully present in whatever we are doing—whether it's engaging in conversation, working on a project, or simply having a meal. Integrating mindfulness into our daily activities allows us to foster a deeper connection to the present moment, cultivating mental clarity, emotional balance, and overall wellbeing. The beauty of mindfulness lies in its versatility—it can be woven into the fabric of everyday life.

Integrating Mindfulness Seamlessly Into Daily Activities

While many people may begin practicing mindfulness during a formal session of meditation or mindful breathing, the real power of mindfulness comes when it is integrated into daily life. The key to incorporating mindfulness throughout your day is understanding that it's not about making dramatic changes, but rather about turning routine actions into moments of awareness.

When you consciously bring your attention to the task at hand, even something as simple as brushing your teeth or folding laundry, you invite mindfulness into that moment. The practice doesn't require elaborate rituals or special techniques—it's about slowing down and paying attention to the here and now. In fact, integrating mindfulness into routine actions can be one of the most effective ways to bring it into your daily life. You can start by simply acknowledging your surroundings, noticing the sensations in your body, and being aware of the act itself.

For instance, while you're eating, try focusing on the taste, texture, and temperature of your food. Instead of rushing through the meal, savor each bite, noticing the experience as it unfolds. The same applies when walking. Instead of thinking about where you're going or what you need to do next, simply pay attention to the act of walking—how your feet feel as they touch the ground, the rhythm of your steps, the sounds around you, and the sensation of air on your skin.

Through these small, intentional actions, you can start to transform routine activities into moments of mindfulness. These moments don't need to be long, but they do need to be deliberate. When you make the choice to be present, you create a stronger sense of connection to both yourself and the world around you.

The Importance of Pausing Throughout the Day

A crucial aspect of cultivating mindful presence is learning how to pause throughout the day. Life can feel full, and we often find ourselves rushing from one task to the next. However, it's during these in-between moments that we can cultivate mindfulness. Pausing, even for a few seconds, to check in with yourself can help restore your focus and bring you back to the present moment.

A simple pause could happen before answering a phone call, before entering a meeting, or even before reacting to something that triggers an emotional response. These pauses allow you to gather your thoughts, center yourself, and assess how you're feeling, both physically and emotionally. By simply noticing what's happening in your body and mind at that moment, you bring awareness to the present.

The value of this pause lies in its ability to interrupt the automatic, habitual flow of actions. When we operate on autopilot, we can easily slip into a pattern of reacting rather than responding consciously. A mindful pause helps us regain control over our thoughts and actions, ensuring that we move through our day with intention.

Mindfulness isn't about perfection; it's about noticing and returning to the present moment without judgment. When you pause to check in with yourself, you are practicing this awareness, and over time, these intentional pauses accumulate, creating a mindful rhythm to your day.

Mindfulness in Everyday Tasks

Mindfulness shines brightest when it's applied to the most mundane and routine activities. It's in these small, everyday tasks that mindfulness can truly enhance our experience of life. These tasks, which often go unnoticed, hold the potential for deep presence and awareness. Whether it's washing dishes, making a cup of tea, or sitting down to work, each of these moments can become a touchstone for mindfulness.

Take eating, for example. Often, we eat quickly and without much attention, distracted by the next task or thought. But when we slow down and bring awareness to the act of eating, we deepen our connection to the food, our bodies, and the nourishment we are receiving. This not only improves our relationship with food but also helps us become more attuned to our body's signals, preventing overeating and promoting better digestion.

The same approach can be applied to work. It's easy to become overwhelmed by a long to-do list, constantly thinking about what's next or rushing to finish tasks. But by being present with each individual task—no matter how small—you can bring more clarity and focus to your work. Instead of worrying about the entire project or multitasking, focus solely on the task at hand. This focused attention allows you to complete your work with greater efficiency and a sense of fulfillment.

Additionally, everyday tasks like walking or even waiting in line can be transformed into mindful moments. Walking becomes an opportunity to feel the ground beneath your feet and appreciate the act of movement. Waiting in line becomes an opportunity to check in with your breath and body, noticing what's happening in your mind without rushing through the moment. By turning these small, routine activities into opportunities for mindfulness, you create a life that is grounded in the present.

Managing Distractions and Regaining Focus

One of the greatest challenges in maintaining mindfulness is managing distractions. It's easy to be pulled away from the present moment by thoughts, emotions, or external stimuli. However, mindfulness offers a powerful tool to help us manage distractions and regain focus.

When you notice that your mind has wandered—whether due to a thought, an emotion, or a distraction—simply observe it without judgment. Rather than getting frustrated or irritated, recognize that distractions are a natural part of the process. The act of noticing your distraction is, in itself, a mindful moment. Once you acknowledge the distraction, gently return your focus to the task or experience at hand.

A helpful strategy for managing distractions is to set intentional reminders throughout the day to check in with your thoughts and feelings. These reminders can be simple cues—like a gentle stretch, a brief pause, or a deep breath—that signal to you to come back to the present moment. Each time you return to the present, you strengthen your ability to focus and deepen your mindfulness practice.

Another way to manage distractions is to reduce external interruptions. While we can't control everything around us, we can create an environment that supports focus and awareness. This may mean setting boundaries with others or eliminating unnecessary distractions during certain tasks. However, mindfulness also teaches us to stay focused and present, even when distractions arise. The key is not to fight against distractions but to gently guide yourself back to the present when they occur.

The Cumulative Effect of Small Mindful Moments

Mindfulness is not about grand gestures or dramatic transformations. Rather, it's about the small, everyday moments of awareness that accumulate over time. When we begin to incorporate mindfulness into even the smallest of tasks—like brushing our teeth or having a conversation—we begin to cultivate a mindset of presence that pervades our entire day.

These small, mindful moments build upon one another, creating a foundation of clarity, calm, and balance. As we bring more awareness to our day-to-day activities, we begin to notice shifts in our mental state and emotional wellbeing. We may find ourselves feeling more centered, less reactive, and more focused.

Over time, these moments of mindfulness can have a profound impact on our overall quality of life. By practicing mindfulness in everyday tasks, we begin to experience life more fully, without being caught in the rush of thoughts, worries, and distractions. We begin to savor each moment, finding richness in the simplicity of our day-to-day experiences.

Being Present

Mindfulness is not a practice confined to specific moments or activities—it's a way of being that can be integrated into every aspect of life. By cultivating mindful presence throughout the day, we can transform routine actions into opportunities for awareness, enhancing our overall wellbeing. Through intentional pauses, focused attention, and the ability to manage distractions, mindfulness offers a path to greater clarity, emotional balance, and mental calm.

Ultimately, mindfulness is about being present—not just in meditation, but in every aspect of life. The more we practice mindfulness in our everyday tasks, the more it becomes a natural part of who we are. And through this, we can experience life with a deeper sense of purpose, focus, and presence.

CHAPTER 14: THE ART OF LETTING GO

In life, we often encounter challenges, discomfort, and a variety of circumstances that trigger strong emotions or thoughts. Whether it's holding onto past regrets, resisting the way things are, or finding it difficult to move forward after a setback, we frequently find ourselves stuck in a cycle of attachment. The idea of letting go can seem elusive or even unsettling, as we may worry about losing control or giving up something that feels important. Yet, the art of letting go is not about relinquishing control entirely or abandoning what we value. Instead, it's about embracing acceptance and releasing the need to hold onto things that no longer serve us.

Letting go is a powerful and transformative practice. It's the act of allowing ourselves to be free from the grip of old habits, limiting beliefs, or past experiences that hinder our growth and wellbeing. This chapter explores the process of letting go and offers strategies for embracing acceptance, which can create space for new possibilities, clarity, and emotional peace.

Understanding the Concept of Letting Go

Letting go involves releasing attachment to things, thoughts, or emotions that prevent us from moving forward. It's important to distinguish that letting go does not mean ignoring or suppressing emotions. Rather, it's about acknowledging them without allowing them to dominate our thoughts or actions. It means accepting the impermanence of life, understanding that all things—both good and bad—are fleeting, and learning to embrace change.

Many of us hold on tightly to the past, whether it's past experiences, relationships, or even our own self-image. These attachments often create mental and emotional clutter that weighs us down, preventing us from fully engaging with the present moment. Letting go is not a one-time act, but rather a continuous practice that helps us move through life with greater ease and clarity.

The Role of Acceptance in Letting Go

Acceptance is a key element in the process of letting go. It is the recognition and acknowledgment that some things are beyond our control, and that we are not defined by our past experiences or the external circumstances of our lives. When we accept something, we stop fighting against it. We stop trying to change what cannot be changed and instead focus on how to navigate the present moment with grace and resilience.

This doesn't mean we resign ourselves to suffering or allow ourselves to stay in situations that are harmful. Acceptance is about making peace with what is, while still striving to create a better future. It's the practice of being at peace with reality, even when it is uncomfortable or challenging. Acceptance allows us to release our resistance, which, in turn, opens up space for healing and growth.

Learning to accept ourselves—our flaws, imperfections, and mistakes—is also an important part of letting go. Many of us struggle with self-criticism or regret over past actions. But the act of accepting ourselves fully, without judgment, allows us to release the weight of guilt or shame that may hold us back. When we accept ourselves, we are better able to move forward and evolve.

Strategies for Letting Go

1. Observe Your Attachments Without Judgment

The first step in letting go is to become aware of what you're holding onto. This requires self-reflection and the ability to observe your thoughts and emotions without judgment. Notice when you're clinging to something—whether it's an idea, a person, a past experience, or even a particular outcome. Recognize the impact these attachments have on your mental and emotional state.

By observing your attachments, you begin to see how they shape your actions and responses. Often, we attach ourselves to things out of fear or insecurity, not realizing how these attachments hinder our growth. Once you are aware of these attachments, you can begin to let them go. The key is to remain compassionate with yourself during this process, acknowledging that it's okay to feel attached, but that it's also possible to release these attachments when they no longer serve you.

2. Practice Self-Compassion

Letting go is not always easy, and it's important to be gentle with yourself throughout the process. Self-compassion involves treating yourself with kindness and understanding when you encounter difficult emotions or experiences. Instead of criticizing yourself for struggling to let go, practice self-compassion by acknowledging that it's natural to have attachments and that it's okay to need time and support in the process of releasing them.

When you practice self-compassion, you allow yourself the space to grieve, to feel, and to heal. You recognize that letting go is a process, not a destination. Over time, this attitude of self-compassion makes it easier to let go of things that no longer align with your values or desires.

3. Create Healthy Boundaries

Sometimes, letting go involves setting boundaries. Whether it's with people, situations, or activities, establishing healthy boundaries helps you preserve your emotional and mental energy. Boundaries allow you to decide what you will and will not accept in your life, and they create the space necessary for you to release what no longer serves you.

Setting boundaries is not about rejecting others; it's about honoring your own needs and values. It can involve saying no to things that drain you, distancing yourself from toxic relationships, or letting go of obligations that no longer align with your priorities. By creating these boundaries, you create a healthier environment for yourself and allow for personal growth and clarity.

4. Release the Need for Control

Much of our attachment stems from a desire to control outcomes. We want to dictate how things should unfold and are often resistant to uncertainty. However, control is an illusion, and trying to control everything only leads to frustration and exhaustion.

Letting go requires us to release the need to control everything and instead learn to trust the process of life. This doesn't mean abandoning responsibility or effort; it means recognizing that there are forces beyond our control and that sometimes, things will unfold in ways we do not expect. By surrendering the need to control every aspect of our lives, we create the space for spontaneity, joy, and growth.

5. Practice Gratitude and Focus on the Present

Another effective strategy for letting go is practicing gratitude. When we focus on what we have right now, instead of what we wish we had or what we've lost, we shift our attention away from attachment and toward appreciation. Gratitude helps us to accept what is and to release our grasp on what could have been.

Focusing on the present moment, rather than dwelling on the past or worrying about the future, also supports the process of letting go. Mindfulness practices that emphasize the present moment help you detach from the stories, expectations, and attachments that keep you stuck. By returning your attention to the here and now, you free yourself from the grip of the past and open yourself to new possibilities.

6. Embrace Change as Part of Life

Finally, one of the most essential strategies for letting go is to embrace change. Change is inevitable, and it's often the source of much of our resistance. However, when we learn to accept that change is a natural part of life, we can approach it with greater openness and resilience.

Instead of fearing change, try to see it as an opportunity for growth and renewal. Life is always in motion, and by accepting that we can never control everything, we open ourselves up to the flow of life and the potential for new experiences. Letting go becomes easier when we shift our mindset from resistance to acceptance.

Letting Go is a Gift

Letting go is a vital practice for personal growth and emotional wellbeing. It's not about losing something valuable, but rather about creating the space for new experiences, clarity, and peace. By embracing acceptance, practicing self-compassion, setting healthy boundaries, and releasing the need for control or perfection, we can move through life with greater ease and resilience.

The process of letting go is ongoing, and it requires patience and kindness. Each step forward, no matter how small, contributes to your overall sense of freedom and peace. Letting go is a gift you give yourself—an invitation to embrace the present moment and trust the unfolding of life.

CHAPTER 15: MINDFUL MOVEMENT, BREATH, AND YOGA FOR HEALTH AND VITALITY

Introduction to Mindful Movement

Mindful movement is the practice of bringing intentional awareness to every step, gesture, and breath as you engage in physical activity. It is not simply about going through the motions or achieving a specific outcome; instead, mindful movement is about being fully present in each moment, aware of the body's sensations, the rhythm of your breath, and the mind's state. Whether you are practicing yoga, walking, or engaging in any form of physical exercise, incorporating mindfulness into movement allows you to cultivate a deeper connection with your body and promote overall well-being.

When we move mindfully, we are not just performing a task. We are experiencing the movement — noticing the subtle shifts in posture, the alignment of joints, and the way the body feels as it stretches, contracts, and flows. This practice invites us to slow down and pay attention, rather than allowing our thoughts to wander or our movements to be automatic. The goal is to focus entirely on the present moment, fostering a sense of calm and clarity that ripples out to other aspects of our lives.

Mindful movement is an invitation to reconnect with your body, as well as with the space around you. By focusing on your breath, posture, and the sensations within the body, you activate the parasympathetic nervous system, which promotes relaxation and helps reduce stress. In a world that often encourages us to rush through tasks, mindful movement offers a refreshing shift, where each motion becomes an opportunity to ground ourselves and experience the world with a clearer, more focused mind.

In this chapter, we will explore how mindful movement — particularly through breath, yoga, and other physical activities such as nature walks— can enhance both physical and mental health. By incorporating mindfulness into your movement practices, you not only boost your physical vitality but also create moments of tranquility and self-awareness that improve your overall quality of life.

The Essential Role of Breath in Mindful Movement

Breath is the cornerstone of mindful movement. Without breath, movement becomes mechanical, disconnected from the body and the present moment. When you focus on your breath during physical activities, you bring awareness and intention to each action. Breathing mindfully transforms any movement into a deeper experience, connecting mind and body and fostering clarity.

The breath has the unique ability to anchor you in the present moment, enabling you to move with more purpose and grace. Whether you're walking, stretching, or engaging in more intense exercise, your breath becomes a guide, ensuring that your movements are steady and controlled. Mindful breathing also helps to reduce tension, improve oxygenation in the body, and promote relaxation.

Pranayma: Yogic Breathwork

One of the most profound ways to deepen your connection to breath is through the yogic breathing practice of pranayama, the art of breath control in yoga. Pranayama is a powerful tool that can enhance mental clarity, reduce stress, and even improve physical performance. Techniques such as deep, diaphragmatic breathing or alternate nostril breathing help you regulate your nervous system, reduce anxiety, and create a sense of calm and presence. The more you practice pranayama, the more you develop a natural rhythm between breath and movement, creating a harmonious flow within your body.

Yoga for Mindful Movement and for Physical and Mental Clarity

Yoga is a holistic practice that combines mindful movement, breath, and awareness. It goes beyond physical postures and becomes a way to cultivate presence, balance, and mental clarity. In yoga, each movement is connected with a breath, creating a flowing sequence that unites the mind and body. By linking breath with motion, yoga helps to create a seamless experience where movement becomes more fluid, and the mind remains focused and grounded.

The beauty of yoga is its adaptability. Whether you are a beginner or experienced practitioner, yoga offers a path to greater body awareness and connection. It encourages mindfulness in every moment, teaching you to notice how your body feels in each posture, without judgment or expectation. Yoga is not about achieving perfect poses but rather about being present and listening to your body as it unfolds.

The Physiological Benefits of Yoga

Yoga offers a comprehensive approach to improving both physical and mental well-being. It is a practice that unites the body, breath, and mind through movement, breathing exercises, and meditation, leading to profound benefits. In this section, we'll explore the key physiological benefits that yoga provides, including how it enhances flexibility, strength, circulation, and overall vitality.

1. Improved Flexibility and Range of Motion

One of the most well-known benefits of yoga is its ability to increase flexibility. Many yoga poses involve stretching and lengthening muscles, which can gradually improve your range of motion. Over time, the regular practice of yoga can help alleviate tightness in muscles and joints, which can occur from sedentary lifestyles or repetitive movements. By focusing on slow, deliberate movements and holding positions for extended periods, yoga allows the body to gradually open up, reducing stiffness and improving overall mobility.

The increase in flexibility that yoga provides isn't just about becoming more limber — it also helps protect against injury. When muscles and joints are more flexible, they are less likely to be strained or injured during other physical activities. This makes yoga an excellent complement to any fitness routine or active lifestyle.

2. Enhanced Strength and Muscle Tone
Yoga is also a powerful way to build strength, particularly in the core, arms, legs, and back. Many yoga poses require you to hold your body weight in various positions, which helps to strengthen muscles. Poses like Downward-Facing Dog, Plank, and Warrior II demand engagement from multiple muscle groups simultaneously, increasing muscle endurance and toning the body.

The strength gained from yoga isn't just about large muscle groups but also about smaller, stabilizing muscles that often go unnoticed in other forms of exercise. Through yoga, you develop functional strength, which supports better posture, balance, and alignment in everyday movements. Moreover, yoga improves muscle coordination, helping to create a more balanced and connected body.

3. Better Posture and Alignment
Yoga encourages mindful awareness of body alignment, which can have lasting effects on posture. The practice teaches you how to align the spine, pelvis, and limbs in a way that minimizes

tension and promotes balance. Over time, this awareness carries over into daily life, helping you maintain better posture whether you're sitting at a desk, walking, or standing.

Improved posture from yoga can alleviate common issues such as back pain, neck tension, and headaches that are often caused by poor alignment. By strengthening the muscles that support the spine and improving awareness of body mechanics, yoga provides a natural way to enhance posture without the need for external aids.

4. Increased Circulation and Blood Flow

Yoga's combination of gentle stretching and deep breathing promotes circulation throughout the body. Many yoga poses improve blood flow to vital organs and extremities, ensuring that nutrients and oxygen are more effectively delivered to tissues. Enhanced circulation also helps flush out toxins from the body, improving overall health and vitality.

In particular, certain yoga poses are known to increase blood flow to the heart and brain. Poses such as inversions (e.g., Shoulder Stand, Downward Dog) encourage the flow of blood toward the upper body, giving the heart a break and promoting better circulation. This can help improve the efficiency of the cardiovascular system and support heart health.

Breathing techniques, or **pranayama**, further enhance circulation by regulating oxygen levels in the blood and improving lung capacity. As you focus on controlled, deep breaths during yoga, the body's ability to distribute oxygen more efficiently increases, which can improve overall cardiovascular and circulatory health.

5. Regulation of the Nervous System

One of yoga's most powerful physiological effects is its ability to regulate the nervous system. The practice of yoga stimulates the parasympathetic nervous system, which is responsible for the body's relaxation response. When the body is in a state of relaxation, blood pressure drops, heart rate slows down, and stress hormones like cortisol are reduced.

Yoga helps counteract the effects of stress by engaging the nervous system in a way that promotes relaxation, calming the mind and body. Breathwork, particularly techniques like **pranayama**, plays a crucial role in this process. Deep, slow breathing activates the vagus nerve, which sends signals to the brain to slow down the heart rate and promote calm.

The balancing effect on the nervous system is especially beneficial for those who experience chronic stress, anxiety, or insomnia. By practicing yoga regularly, you can strengthen your body's ability to handle stress and maintain a sense of equilibrium even in challenging situations.

6. Enhanced Respiratory Function

Yoga's emphasis on mindful breathing has a direct impact on respiratory function. Pranayama, the art of breath control, encourages deep, diaphragmatic breathing, which can improve lung capacity, increase oxygen intake, and reduce shallow, chest-based breathing patterns that are common during stressful moments.

The practice of intentional breathing in yoga, promotes stronger, more efficient lung function. Regular practice of yogic breathing techniques can help expand lung capacity and improve the effectiveness of oxygen exchange. As a result, you may find that your endurance increases in other physical activities, as your body becomes more efficient at utilizing oxygen.

Yoga also helps regulate the breath during physical exertion. By syncing breath with movement, you develop a natural rhythm that keeps your energy levels balanced and prevents the body from becoming overly fatigued. This connection between breath and movement can enhance performance in yoga as well as other forms of exercise.

7. Mobility and Joint Health

Yoga's low-impact movements when performed correctly tend

to be gentle on the joints, making it an excellent practice for maintaining joint health and flexibility throughout life. Yoga offers a gentle way to move and stretch without putting undue stress on the body. Regular practice helps improve joint mobility, and reduce stiffness. It can help prevent injuries caused by lack of movement or overuse.

8. Boosted Immune System

Yoga stimulates the lymphatic system, which plays a key role in detoxifying the body. Certain poses, such as twists and forward bends, help to stimulate the flow of lymph, flushing out toxins and promoting a cleaner, more vibrant system. The physical movement combined with breathwork enhances circulation and supports the elimination of waste products from the body.

Yoga promotes relaxation and reduces chronic stress, both of which have positive effects on the immune system. By reducing levels of cortisol, the stress hormone, yoga helps to lower inflammation in the body, which in turn supports immune function. As yoga encourages deep breathing, it also stimulates the flow of oxygen and nutrients throughout the body, helping to strengthen the immune system and fight off infections.

In addition, yoga improves sleep quality, which is another factor in maintaining a healthy immune system. When the body is well-rested, it has a better ability to repair and regenerate, which boosts overall health and immunity.

Incorporating Yoga Into Your Routine

Yoga is a multifaceted practice that offers a wide range of physiological benefits. From increased flexibility and strength to enhanced circulation, improved posture, and a regulated nervous system, yoga provides a natural, holistic approach to better health. It connects the mind, body, and breath in a way that supports the body's natural healing processes while also promoting relaxation and mental clarity.

Incorporating yoga into your routine — even for just a few minutes a day — can help foster a deeper connection to your body, reduce stress, improve posture, and enhance overall physical vitality. Whether you are looking to improve strength, flexibility, or simply cultivate a sense of calm and well-being, yoga offers a pathway to a healthier, more balanced life.

Creating a Routine of Mindful Movement

To experience the full benefits of mindful movement, it's helpful to establish a regular practice. Whether you prefer yoga or another form of physical activity, make it a daily or weekly habit. Even 10 to 20 minutes of yoga, combined with mindful breathing, can yield profound effects on your body and mind.

Incorporating pranayama into your routine can also deepen your practice. Set aside time each day for focused breathwork, whether it's at the start or end of your yoga practice or as a separate session. Pranayama can help you manage stress, improve focus, and increase energy, creating a solid foundation for both physical and emotional well-being.

If yoga isn't your primary form of exercise, try adding mindful breathing to your daily activities. Whether you're stretching in the morning, taking a walk, or participating in any physical activity, incorporate breath awareness to bring more presence to the task. Mindful movement doesn't require a mat or formal structure — it's about creating a space for awareness and intentionality in whatever activity you engage in.

CHAPTER 16: OVERCOMING CHALLENGES WITH MINDFULNESS

The Role of Mindfulness in Facing Challenges

Challenges are an inevitable part of life. However, how we respond to them is within our control. Mindfulness teaches us to step back from our immediate reactions and approach difficulties with a sense of awareness and perspective. Instead of being caught up in the whirlwind of emotions and thoughts that challenges often bring, mindfulness encourages us to pause, breathe, and examine the situation from a calm, centered place.

Life is full of challenges—some large, some small. We all encounter obstacles that can cause stress, frustration, and uncertainty. Whether we face difficulties in our personal lives, work, or relationships, challenges often make us feel overwhelmed and out of control. The way we approach and handle these challenges has a profound impact on our overall well-being. Mindfulness, the practice of being fully present and aware in the moment, offers powerful tools for navigating these tough situations with calm, clarity, and resilience. This chapter explores how mindfulness can help us overcome the challenges we face, empowering us to handle difficulties with greater ease and understanding.

In many cases, when we encounter a challenge, our minds begin to race with worry, self-doubt, or fear. We may start to ruminate on worst-case scenarios or imagine outcomes that have yet to occur. This kind of mental habit can exacerbate stress, leaving us feeling helpless and overwhelmed. Mindfulness breaks this cycle by encouraging us to observe our thoughts without judgment. We can acknowledge these emotions and thoughts without letting them control us. By becoming aware of how we are feeling and thinking in the moment, we can make conscious choices about how we respond to the challenge, instead of reacting impulsively.

Cultivating Emotional Awareness

One of the key benefits of mindfulness in overcoming challenges is its ability to enhance emotional awareness. In times of difficulty, we may experience a wide range of emotions— fear, anger, frustration, sadness, or even confusion. Often, we try to avoid or suppress these emotions because they feel uncomfortable. However, mindfulness teaches us to approach these emotions with acceptance and curiosity.

Instead of pushing emotions away, mindfulness encourages us to experience them fully. This doesn't mean acting on them impulsively, but rather allowing ourselves to feel the emotion without judgment. For example, if we feel angry about a difficult situation, mindfulness invites us to observe the anger without attaching a story or label to it. We can notice where we feel the anger in our body, what sensations arise, and how our thoughts might be influencing our emotional experience.

By cultivating emotional awareness, mindfulness allows us to respond more thoughtfully to challenges. We may find that our initial reactions of frustration or anger are not as intense when we acknowledge them and allow them to pass. We can then choose more constructive ways to handle the situation, such as taking a moment to breathe or stepping back to gain perspective before responding.

Staying Present Amidst Uncertainty

Challenges often bring a sense of uncertainty or unpredictability, and uncertainty can trigger anxiety. When we face a situation that feels unfamiliar or outside our control, it is easy to become consumed by worry about the future or regret about the past. Mindfulness offers a way to ground ourselves in the present moment, rather than getting lost in what-ifs or what-could-have-beens.

In times of uncertainty, mindfulness invites us to focus on what is directly in front of us. It reminds us that we cannot control every aspect of the future, but we can control how we respond in the present moment. Whether it's a difficult decision, an unexpected change, or a challenging project, staying present helps us approach the situation with clarity and focus. Rather than fixating on what may or may not happen, we can take each moment as it comes, handling what is before us without becoming overwhelmed by what lies ahead.

Developing Patience and Acceptance

Patience is an essential quality when dealing with challenges. Often, we want problems to be solved immediately, and the longer they persist, the more frustrated we become. Mindfulness teaches us to practice patience by encouraging us to accept the present moment as it is, without the need to rush or force an outcome.

Mindfulness invites us to embrace the ebb and flow of life's challenges with a sense of patience and understanding. It allows us to step back from the urge to push through every obstacle and instead move through the situation with calm awareness. This does not mean passivity or resignation, but rather cultivating an attitude of acceptance toward the process. When we accept that challenges take time and effort, we free ourselves from the burden of trying to force an immediate resolution, and in doing so, we reduce stress and anxiety.

Along with patience comes acceptance. Acceptance does not mean that we agree with or like the situation at hand, but that we recognize it as part of our reality in the present moment. By accepting the challenge, we stop fighting against it and allow ourselves the space to deal with it as it is. This shift in mindset makes it easier to engage with the challenge in a constructive way, instead of resisting or avoiding it.

Cultivating Problem-Solving Skills

Mindfulness is not just about observing challenges but also about developing effective ways to handle them. When we approach problems with mindfulness, we can enhance our problem-solving abilities. Instead of reacting impulsively or becoming paralyzed by anxiety, we can take a calm, methodical approach to find solutions.

Mindful problem-solving involves recognizing our emotions and thoughts, understanding the situation clearly, and then taking measured steps to address the issue. Rather than jumping into a solution out of urgency, mindfulness encourages us to pause and reflect. This pause allows us to consider various options, assess the situation from different angles, and choose the course of action that feels most aligned with our values and goals.

By applying mindfulness to problem-solving, we are more likely to find creative solutions, make thoughtful decisions, and avoid rash choices that may lead to regret later. This practice helps us approach challenges with a sense of confidence and clarity, knowing that we have the ability to handle whatever comes our way.

Moving Forward with Confidence

Overcoming challenges with mindfulness is not about avoiding difficulty but about approaching life's hurdles with a mindset of confidence and equanimity. Mindfulness enables us to face obstacles with an inner strength that comes from being grounded in the present moment. We learn to see challenges as part of the process, rather than as insurmountable barriers.

When we practice mindfulness, we tap into a deep reservoir of resilience, patience, and awareness that helps us navigate even the most difficult situations. We are able to respond with clarity and balance, reducing the impact of stress and anxiety on our mental and emotional well-being. Through mindful engagement, we become more confident in our ability to handle challenges, knowing that we have the tools to meet them with presence, patience, and grace.

The Role of Perspective in Facing Challenges

Mindfulness also encourages us to shift our perspective when facing challenges. When we are caught up in difficulty, it is easy to view the situation as insurmountable or overwhelming. We may see it as an obstacle that defines us or as a source of constant stress. Mindfulness helps us step back and view challenges as temporary situations, not permanent realities.

This shift in perspective allows us to see the bigger picture. We realize that every challenge, no matter how daunting it may seem, is just a part of the greater flow of life. By maintaining this perspective, we can reduce the pressure we place on ourselves to "fix" everything immediately and instead approach challenges with a sense of curiosity and acceptance. This mindset enables us to grow through adversity and find meaning in even the most difficult experiences.

Moreover, when we adopt a mindful perspective, we are less likely to catastrophize a situation. We learn to see challenges for what they truly are—difficult, yes, but also opportunities for personal growth and development. This perspective can change our entire relationship with challenges, transforming them from something to avoid into something we can face with strength and clarity.

Developing Compassion for Ourselves

As we face challenges, it is important to be compassionate with ourselves. Mindfulness teaches us that we don't have to be perfect or have all the answers. Instead of being harsh or critical of ourselves during difficult times, mindfulness encourages self-compassion. This involves treating ourselves with the same kindness and understanding that we would offer to a friend facing adversity.

By practicing self-compassion, we give ourselves permission to experience challenges without judgment. We accept that it's okay to struggle, and that we don't need to be flawless in our responses. This compassionate mindset fosters resilience, as we are able to bounce back more easily when we are kind to ourselves in the face of hardship. We recognize that self-compassion is a vital part of our healing process, allowing us to move through challenges with grace and self-awareness.

Mindfulness to Overcome

Mindfulness provides us with the essential tools to overcome life's challenges with calm and clarity. By becoming more aware of our thoughts, emotions, and reactions, we can develop a more balanced approach to adversity. Through mindfulness, we cultivate resilience, emotional awareness, patience, and problem-solving skills—all of which empower us to face challenges with greater confidence. Whether we are dealing with everyday difficulties or larger obstacles, mindfulness allows us to remain grounded and centered, turning challenges into opportunities for growth and learning. By embracing mindfulness in difficult times, we not only enhance our ability to overcome challenges but also cultivate a deeper sense of inner strength and peace.

Through mindful practice, we begin to recognize that challenges are a natural part of life's journey. Rather than shying away from them, we can embrace them as opportunities to strengthen our resilience, expand our emotional awareness, and deepen our understanding of ourselves. With mindfulness, we have the power to transform how we engage with life's difficulties—turning each challenge into a chance for growth, learning, and self-discovery.

CHAPTER 17: THE CALMING EFFECT OF MINDFULNESS

Calm is a quality that brings peace to both the mind and body, offering clarity and tranquility even in the most challenging moments. It's a state of being that we can cultivate, regardless of the circumstances around us. Through mindfulness, we can learn to bring calm into our lives, allowing us to feel steady and peaceful even amid life's complexities.

Mindfulness teaches us to focus on the present moment, offering a way to connect with what is happening right now, without the distractions of the past or future. This practice of being present helps foster a deep sense of calm that can carry us through various experiences, whether they are peaceful or more demanding. In this chapter, we explore how mindfulness can help us increase calm, stay grounded, and respond to challenges with greater ease and clarity.

How Mindfulness Cultivates Calm

Mindfulness begins with the simple act of paying attention to the present moment. In doing so, we step away from the constant flow of thoughts, worries, and distractions that can often feel overwhelming. By focusing on the here and now, we free ourselves from the pressures of past regrets or future anxieties, which often prevent us from experiencing the peace that is available in the present.

When we practice mindfulness, we can bring our attention to

the small, subtle moments in our lives that are easy to overlook. Whether it's the feeling of our breath entering and leaving our body, the sensation of the ground beneath our feet, or the sound of a gentle breeze, mindfulness invites us to connect with these moments, helping us to feel anchored in the present. This simple act of focusing on what is happening in the now creates a feeling of stillness and calm, allowing us to experience life with a sense of ease.

Mindfulness also encourages us to notice our thoughts and emotions without being swept away by them. Instead of being caught up in an ongoing stream of thoughts, we learn to observe them as they arise, letting them pass naturally without attaching to them. This approach helps reduce the intensity of emotional reactions, allowing us to maintain a sense of calm even when our minds are busy or our feelings are strong.

Staying Grounded in Calm

One of the greatest benefits of mindfulness is its ability to help us stay grounded in calm, even during difficult or chaotic moments. Life doesn't always offer the serenity we might wish for, but mindfulness allows us to find stillness within, no matter the circumstances. When we are grounded in calm, we are better able to respond to challenges with clarity and resilience, rather than becoming overwhelmed.

A simple practice to stay grounded is focusing on the breath. The breath is always with us, providing a natural anchor when we feel ourselves becoming unsteady. By bringing our attention to the rhythm of our breathing, we can help calm the mind and body. With each breath, we connect with the present moment, allowing our thoughts and emotions to settle. This simple but powerful practice brings us back to a state of tranquility.

Additionally, mindfulness encourages us to notice our body's sensations. If we feel anxious or restless, we can tune in to how our body feels in the moment. Perhaps we notice the weight of our body on the chair, the sensation of our feet on the floor, or the gentle movement of our muscles as we breathe. By grounding ourselves in these physical sensations, we become more anchored in the present moment and less likely to be overwhelmed by external stresses or internal turbulence.

Embracing the Present Moment

One of the most effective ways mindfulness helps us cultivate calm is by drawing our attention to the present moment. When we focus on what is directly in front of us, we take the pressure off our minds to anticipate or worry about the future. Mindfulness invites us to let go of past regrets or future anxieties and simply be with what is happening right now.

This practice can be applied to any part of our day, whether we are eating, walking, or even simply sitting still. By bringing our full attention to whatever task is before us, we create a sense of peace. When we are fully engaged in the present moment, we stop looking for distractions or sources of stress. We become more aware of the small, calming details of life that are often overlooked, such as the taste of food, the sound of rain, or the warmth of the sun. These simple moments of mindfulness connect us to the stillness that is always available.

Even in the midst of chaos, mindfulness allows us to remain anchored in the present moment. When we pause and breathe, we center ourselves, allowing any turbulence to pass without throwing us off balance. The more we practice this, the easier it becomes to maintain calmness in situations where we might otherwise feel frazzled.

Mindfulness and Anxiety

Anxiety often arises when we feel threatened by uncertainty or the unknown. It can cause the mind to race, conjuring up worst-case scenarios or exaggerated fears. This flood of anxious thoughts can overwhelm us, making it difficult to focus or make clear decisions. Anxiety has a way of amplifying fear and tension, creating a sense of unease that seems to pervade every part of our experience.

Mindfulness can offer a way to help manage our anxiety by encouraging us to disengage from overwhelming thoughts and return to the present moment. When we practice mindfulness, we learn to notice the anxious thoughts without becoming entangled in them. Instead of allowing them to dictate our feelings or actions, mindfulness encourages us to observe these thoughts with curiosity and awareness.

By acknowledging the presence of anxiety—without trying to push it away or change it—we create space between ourselves and the emotion. We can recognize it as just a feeling, not something that defines us or controls us. Through this act of awareness, anxiety starts to lose its grip. It is no longer an overpowering force but something we can see, understand, and move through.

Using mindfulness to observe anxiety rather than react to it can help to reduce its intensity. With time, we develop the ability to face anxious moments with greater calm and perspective, knowing that anxiety is a natural response but one that we don't have to let dominate our lives. Through mindfulness, we reclaim the peace that resides within us, no matter the circumstances.

Mindfulness helps us shift from reacting to our anxiety to responding with calm. When we feel anxious, we can ground ourselves by focusing on our breath or tuning into our body's sensations. This helps interrupt the cycle of worry and brings us back to a steady, balanced state. Instead of being overwhelmed by what-ifs or imagined fears, mindfulness brings us back to what is happening right now, allowing us to feel more present and in control.

The Calming Power of Observation

Mindfulness offers a powerful way to connect with our internal experiences by observing them without the need to change them. This approach allows us to acknowledge how we are feeling, what we are thinking, or what sensations we are experiencing, without the urge to manipulate or fix anything.

Instead of becoming reactive to our experiences, we simply observe them with curiosity.

For example, if we feel a surge of frustration, mindfulness encourages us to notice the sensation of frustration in our body. Where do we feel it? Is it in our chest? Our stomach? What does it feel like? Through this process of observation, the emotion begins to lose its intensity. We start to realize that emotions are not permanent—they come and go, and by observing them with presence, we allow them to pass naturally. This shift in perspective helps us stay calm, even when the emotional tides seem strong.

Mindfulness also helps us connect with the impermanence of our thoughts. Thoughts may arise, but they do not have to define our experience or influence our actions. By practicing mindfulness, we can develop a deeper awareness of how thoughts move through our minds and let them go without attachment. This makes it easier to stay calm, as we realize that thoughts are simply mental events—temporary and passing.

Mindfulness For Greater Calm and Perspective

Mindfulness is a practice that empowers us to cultivate calmness and clarity in our lives. By being fully present and aware of our thoughts, emotions, and physical sensations, we can tap into a deep sense of peace that helps us navigate even the most challenging situations. Rather than becoming overwhelmed by our reactions or the demands of life, mindfulness encourages us to slow down, take a breath, and center ourselves.

Through mindfulness, we develop the ability to stay grounded, even when things around us feel unsettled. We learn that calm is not a distant, elusive state but something we can create and access at any time. Whether through the simple act of focusing on our breath, tuning in to our body's sensations, or observing our internal experience, mindfulness helps us remain centered and steady, bringing greater calm and perspective to our lives.

With continued practice, we can cultivate an inner tranquility that remains with us, no matter what life throws our way.

CHAPTER 18: OVERCOMING PERFECTIONISM WITH MINDFULNESS

The Weight of Perfectionism

Perfectionism, often celebrated as a pursuit of excellence, can instead act as an unwieldy burden, making it difficult to enjoy our achievements or feel at peace with ourselves. This constant striving for flawlessness tends to make us fixate on minor details, rarely feeling satisfied with the results, no matter how much effort we invest. While ambition and high standards are not inherently negative, the pursuit of perfection can lead to stress, dissatisfaction, and burnout. In its extreme form, it robs us of the ability to appreciate our own progress, pushing us to focus on what's missing or what's wrong instead of recognizing what has been accomplished.

Mindfulness, a practice of being present and aware in each moment, offers a transformative approach to overcoming perfectionism. By encouraging us to embrace imperfection, mindfulness allows us to shift our focus from striving for an unattainable standard to accepting ourselves as we are, flaws and all. Through mindfulness, we can learn to respond to our tendencies toward perfectionism with patience, self-compassion, and a sense of balance. This chapter explores how mindfulness can be a powerful tool in managing and overcoming perfectionism, offering a path to greater self-acceptance and peace.

The Pressure of Perfectionism

At its core, perfectionism arises from the desire to avoid failure or criticism. The internal dialogue of a perfectionist is often harsh and unrelenting, demanding that everything be "just right" or "perfect." This drive to meet an impossible standard can lead to feelings of inadequacy when those standards inevitably fall short. The weight of perfectionism often manifests in both personal and professional life, from overly critical self-evaluations to the fear of making mistakes or appearing vulnerable in front of others. This constant internal pressure can lead to anxiety, self-doubt, and a tendency to overwork in an effort to prove one's worth or achieve an ideal.

In relationships, perfectionism can cause tension, as the desire to meet others' expectations or present an idealized version of oneself leads to a lack of authentic connection. We may push ourselves to always be "on" and perform at our best, neglecting the parts of ourselves that are less polished or "imperfect." This can result in feelings of loneliness or disconnection, even in the company of loved ones, as we focus more on presenting an image than on building a genuine bond.

Mindfulness offers a reprieve from this cycle of self-criticism. By practicing mindfulness, we develop a healthier relationship with our own expectations. Rather than constantly focusing on what's missing or what needs to be better, mindfulness teaches us to appreciate the present moment and recognize the effort we are putting forth, regardless of the outcome. It allows us to see that imperfection is part of being human, and that it's okay to make mistakes or not have everything figured out. This shift in mindset helps reduce the internal pressure that perfectionism creates, opening the door to greater peace and acceptance.

The Role of Mindfulness in Embracing Imperfection

Mindfulness teaches us to observe our thoughts and feelings

without getting attached to them. This quality is particularly important in dealing with perfectionism, as the perfectionist's mind tends to fixate on thoughts of failure, judgment, or inadequacy. Through mindfulness, we can observe these thoughts as they arise without identifying with them. Rather than letting them dictate our actions, we can see them as temporary experiences—thoughts that come and go, without the need to give them power or let them shape our self-worth.

One of the first steps in overcoming perfectionism with mindfulness is learning to accept imperfection. When we are mindful, we recognize that imperfection is an inherent part of life. No task, no project, and no person is truly perfect, and that's not only okay but also natural. Mindfulness encourages us to embrace these imperfections as part of the process rather than seeing them as failures. Instead of focusing on flaws, we begin to value the journey—the effort, growth, and learning that happens along the way.

This shift toward embracing imperfection can be liberating. When we stop expecting ourselves to be flawless, we free ourselves from the constraints of perfectionism. We can take a deep breath and acknowledge that it's acceptable to not have everything under control. It's in the moments of imperfection that growth occurs, and mindfulness teaches us to be present with that process, rather than fixating on the end result.

Self-Compassion: The Antidote to Perfectionism

A key element of mindfulness is self-compassion—the ability to treat ourselves with the same kindness, patience, and understanding that we would offer to a friend in need. Perfectionism often thrives on self-criticism, where we are our harshest critics. Instead of giving ourselves grace when things don't go as planned, we may judge ourselves with an unyielding inner voice, reinforcing the idea that we must always do better.

Self-compassion, supported by mindfulness, challenges this inner dialogue. When we practice self-compassion, we allow ourselves to be human. We acknowledge that we will make mistakes, miss the mark, and fall short of expectations from time to time, and that this is not only acceptable but part of the human experience. Through mindfulness, we learn to quiet the critical voice inside us and replace it with one of gentleness and understanding. This compassionate perspective softens the impact of imperfection, allowing us to move through challenges without the burden of harsh judgment.

Self-compassion in the context of mindfulness is not about lowering standards or excusing poor behavior, but rather about approaching ourselves with understanding when we inevitably encounter setbacks. Rather than beating ourselves up for not achieving perfection, we can gently remind ourselves that mistakes are opportunities for learning and growth. This mindset shift helps us approach challenges with resilience, rather than retreating in fear of failure.

Letting Go of Unrealistic Standards

Perfectionism is often driven by unrealistic standards—ideas about how things should be that are not grounded in reality. These expectations are typically rooted in the desire to impress others, avoid criticism, or gain approval. However, these standards often do not reflect what is truly important or what is attainable. They are artificial constructs that create constant stress and dissatisfaction.

Mindfulness helps us detach from these unrealistic standards by teaching us to focus on the present moment rather than fixating on external outcomes. When we practice mindfulness, we begin to notice the mental patterns that lead us to set excessively high standards or pursue unattainable goals. We become more aware of how these unrealistic expectations affect our well-being and how they might lead to feelings of disappointment or frustration when we inevitably fall short.

By cultivating mindfulness, we can begin to let go of the need for perfection. We can set more realistic, achievable goals that are aligned with our values and what truly matters. Mindfulness allows us to define success on our own terms—based on effort, progress, and growth—rather than on unattainable ideals or external validation. This not only reduces stress but also helps us approach tasks with a greater sense of purpose and fulfillment.

Mindful Practices to Overcome Perfectionism

Mindful practices can be a powerful way to combat perfectionism and cultivate a healthier relationship with ourselves. One such practice is to pause and take a breath whenever we feel the urge to push for perfection. By simply taking a moment to breathe, we allow ourselves to step out of the cycle of striving and tune into the present moment. This can help create space to observe our feelings without judgment and make more conscious choices about how to move forward.

Another helpful practice is to set small, realistic goals rather than overwhelming ourselves with grand, perfectionistic expectations. By breaking tasks into manageable steps, we can focus on the process rather than obsessing over the end result. This approach encourages us to appreciate the journey, rather than fixating on the destination, and fosters a sense of accomplishment along the way.

Finally, practicing gratitude can also help shift our focus away from the pursuit of perfection. By taking time each day to reflect on what we are grateful for, we reframe our perspective from what's lacking or imperfect to what's already good and sufficient. This simple practice can help diminish the power of perfectionism and remind us of the many positive aspects of our lives, even when things are not "perfect."

Embracing Imperfection with Mindfulness

Perfectionism can be a heavy burden, one that robs us of joy, peace, and self-acceptance. Mindfulness offers a path to breaking free from the cycle of self-criticism and unattainable standards by fostering a sense of presence, acceptance, and self-compassion. Through mindfulness, we learn to embrace imperfection as a natural and valuable part of life, rather than something to avoid or fear.

By practicing mindfulness, we let go of unrealistic expectations and create space for self-acceptance and growth. We can approach life with greater ease, confidence, and a deeper appreciation for the process rather than the outcome. In doing so, we cultivate a sense of peace that comes from knowing we are enough, just as we are.

Mindfulness helps us face our challenges with a renewed sense of clarity and compassion, making it easier to let go of perfectionism and live more fully in the present moment.

CHAPTER 19: FOSTERING RESILIENCE THROUGH MINDFULNESS

Mindfulness and Resilience: Building Inner Strength Through Awareness

Resilience is the ability to remain steady and composed when life presents its most challenging moments. It is not simply about enduring hardship but about navigating it with clarity, emotional strength, and the capacity to adapt. Resilient people don't avoid difficulties; instead, they find a way to move through them while maintaining their sense of balance and well-being. In moments of adversity, resilience provides a foundation that allows us to respond thoughtfully, rather than react impulsively or with fear.

Mindfulness, the practice of staying fully aware and present in the moment, is an invaluable tool in fostering this kind of resilience. When we approach difficult situations with mindfulness, we become more attuned to our internal experiences—our thoughts, emotions, and bodily sensations. This awareness allows us to respond with a clear mind and an open heart, giving us the ability to adapt and find stability, even in moments of chaos. Through mindfulness, we not only develop resilience but also a deeper sense of inner strength that helps us face life's uncertainties with greater confidence and composure.

Characteristics of Resilience

Resilience is often thought of as a person's ability to withstand hardship and recover from setbacks. However, true resilience goes beyond simply bouncing back from adversity; it involves the capacity to grow and learn from difficult experiences. Resilient individuals are not immune to pain or stress, but they are able to adapt, find meaning, and maintain a sense of balance in the midst of challenges. They have a deep sense of inner strength, and their emotional flexibility allows them to cope with life's difficulties in a healthy and constructive manner.

Several key characteristics define resilience:

1. **Emotional Awareness**: Resilient individuals are in tune with their emotions. They do not suppress or ignore their feelings but acknowledge them and respond in a way that is measured and intentional.

2. **Adaptability**: Resilience involves the ability to adjust to changing circumstances, particularly when faced with uncertainty or difficult situations. Resilient individuals are flexible, able to accept new realities and find ways to adapt without losing their sense of self.

3. **Optimism and Hope**: Although resilience does not mean ignoring challenges, resilient individuals tend to maintain a positive outlook, even when times are tough. They trust that difficult moments are temporary and that they have the strength to overcome them.

4. **Perseverance**: Resilience is characterized by the ability to keep going, even when the road ahead is difficult. Resilient individuals do not give up easily; they understand that persistence is key to overcoming

adversity.

5. **Self-Compassion**: Resilient individuals are kind to themselves in times of struggle. They do not criticize themselves for feeling vulnerable or for facing difficulties. Instead, they recognize that setbacks are a normal part of life, and they treat themselves with understanding and care.

Mindfulness fosters each of these characteristics of resilience. By promoting awareness, presence, and acceptance, mindfulness enables us to cultivate emotional awareness, adaptability, optimism, perseverance, and self-compassion—all essential qualities for resilience.

Mindfulness and Building Resilience

Mindfulness is an effective tool for building resilience because it helps us develop the awareness and presence necessary to navigate difficult circumstances with clarity and balance. When we are mindful, we become more attuned to our thoughts, feelings, and bodily sensations, which allows us to respond to stressors in a more thoughtful and intentional way, rather than reacting impulsively or emotionally.

In moments of difficulty, mindfulness teaches us to focus on what is within our control. Instead of getting overwhelmed by the situation or imagining worst-case scenarios, mindfulness encourages us to stay grounded in the present moment. This practice helps us to recognize that, while we may not be able to control the circumstances we face, we can control how we respond to them.

One of the key ways that mindfulness fosters resilience is by promoting emotional regulation. When we encounter stress or adversity, it is natural for our emotions to become heightened. Fear, anger, sadness, and frustration can take over, making it difficult to think clearly or make sound decisions. Mindfulness allows us to pause and observe these emotions without becoming consumed by them. By observing our feelings without attachment or judgment, we create space between ourselves and our emotions, which helps us maintain a sense of control and perspective.

This space allows us to choose how to respond to adversity. We may feel fear or sadness, but we do not need to let those emotions dictate our behavior. Instead, mindfulness enables us to respond with calmness, patience, and understanding, which builds our emotional strength and resilience.

Navigating Uncertainty and Change

Life is full of uncertainty and change, and how we handle these aspects of life often determines our level of resilience. When things feel unstable or unpredictable, it is easy to become anxious or overwhelmed. Mindfulness offers us a way to stay centered, even when we are faced with uncertainty. By focusing on the present moment, we are able to remain anchored, rather than getting swept away by worry about the future or regret about the past.

When we practice mindfulness in the face of change, we learn to approach uncertainty with curiosity and openness, rather than fear. Instead of resisting change or wishing things were different, mindfulness encourages us to accept the reality of the present moment. This acceptance does not mean passivity; rather, it means acknowledging the situation as it is and finding ways to move forward with a calm and balanced mindset.

Mindfulness helps us see that change is inevitable, and that it is not something to fear or resist, but something we can adapt to and navigate with resilience. In moments of change, we can use mindfulness to reconnect with ourselves, find our center, and take each moment as it comes, without getting caught up in the anxiety of what might happen next.

Staying Grounded and Focused in Turbulent Times

Turbulent times—whether they involve personal struggles, societal upheaval, or external crises—can leave us feeling unsettled and uncertain. In these moments, mindfulness provides a grounding force that helps us maintain a sense of stability and clarity. Instead of becoming overwhelmed by chaos, mindfulness teaches us to stay present and focused on the task at hand, one step at a time.

In times of stress, it can be easy to become scattered, with our thoughts racing in every direction. Mindfulness helps us bring our attention back to the present, allowing us to stay focused and make decisions with a clear mind. By practicing mindfulness, we can avoid getting lost in worry or distraction, and instead direct our energy toward finding solutions and taking practical action.

One of the key ways mindfulness helps us stay grounded during turbulent times is by fostering acceptance. When we face difficulty or uncertainty, our first instinct may be to resist or fight against the situation. However, mindfulness encourages us to accept what is happening in the present moment, without judgment or resistance. This acceptance creates a sense of peace and calm, even in the midst of chaos. It allows us to move through difficult times with a sense of grace, knowing that we are not fighting against the current, but instead navigating it with resilience and strength.

Mindfulness as a Source of Stability and Clarity

In moments of chaos, mindfulness offers us a sense of stability and clarity that allows us to make decisions and act with confidence. When we are fully present and aware, we can see the situation for what it truly is, without the distortion of fear, anxiety, or other emotional reactions. This clarity enables us to make decisions that are aligned with our values and priorities, rather than reacting impulsively or out of fear.

By staying grounded in the present moment, we are able to gain perspective on the situation at hand. This perspective helps us see that, even in the face of adversity, we have the strength and resilience to move forward. Mindfulness allows us to access our inner resources, drawing upon our capacity for calm, focus, and adaptability in times of challenge.

Developing Inner Strength Through Mindfulness

Mindfulness is a powerful tool for building resilience, helping us respond to adversity with emotional strength, adaptability, and clarity. By fostering awareness of our thoughts, feelings, and bodily sensations, mindfulness allows us to navigate challenges with a calm, grounded mindset. In moments of stress, uncertainty, and change, mindfulness provides us with the tools to stay present, focused, and resilient, enabling us to handle life's difficulties with grace and strength.

Resilience is not about avoiding challenges, but about facing them with a sense of inner strength and balance. Mindfulness helps us cultivate this inner strength, offering us the clarity and perspective to navigate even the most turbulent times. Through mindfulness, we can develop the emotional resilience necessary to not only survive adversity but thrive in the face of it, emerging stronger, wiser, and more capable than before.

CHAPTER 20: MINDFULNESS TO COMBAT INTRUSIVE THOUGHTS

Dealing with Intrusive Thoughts: Sending Them Out of Our Minds

Intrusive thoughts are uninvited mental events that can disrupt our sense of calm and focus. These thoughts often arise unexpectedly, and they can range from fleeting worries to more persistent, unsettling ideas. Sometimes, they seem to come out of nowhere, and no matter how much we try to ignore them, they seem to hang around. They can be negative, irrational, or even absurd, and they can cause stress or discomfort, especially when we try to force them away.

One of the core teachings of mindfulness is that thoughts are transient and do not define us. They come and go, and we are not obligated to engage with them or let them dictate our emotional state. In the face of intrusive thoughts, mindfulness offers us the opportunity to observe these thoughts from a distance, recognizing that they are simply passing mental events. By acknowledging that they are just thoughts and not facts, we free ourselves from their grip.

When an intrusive thought arises, mindfulness allows us to create space between ourselves and the thought. Instead of reacting to it or following it down a path of worry or rumination, we can choose to let it pass. One way to do this is by visualizing the thought as something that can be sent out of your mind. You can imagine the thought as an object—like a balloon or a leaf—that is easily carried away by the breeze. With this simple image, you give yourself permission to let go of the thought, watching it drift further and further away until it no longer holds any power over you.

This process doesn't require force or suppression; it's about creating the space to release the thought without getting caught up in it. The more we practice this, the easier it becomes to detach from such thoughts, no longer feeling the need to wrestle with them. Instead, we allow them to pass by, letting them fade into the background as we return our focus to the present moment.

This practice of sending thoughts out can also be viewed as a way of restoring balance and order in our minds. When we feel overwhelmed by a particular thought, it can help to pause and acknowledge it, but then consciously decide to release it. This could be done by imagining the thought moving out of our awareness—like an object that no longer serves a purpose. This doesn't mean we ignore or suppress it, but rather that we recognize it as something temporary that we don't need to carry with us.

By using mindfulness to release intrusive thoughts, we free ourselves from the cycle of rumination and self-criticism. We recognize that thoughts come and go, and we have the ability to let go of those that no longer serve us. This process of letting go can help us return to a state of mental clarity, where we can engage more fully with the present moment, free from the weight of unnecessary mental clutter.

Over time, with practice, sending thoughts out of our minds becomes a natural skill. The more we practice releasing intrusive thoughts, the less power they have over us. We become better at choosing which thoughts to engage with and which ones to allow to pass by. This ability to detach from disruptive thoughts creates space for new, more constructive thinking patterns and brings a sense of inner peace and resilience. We learn to trust ourselves in managing our mental landscape, knowing we can return to a place of calm and presence at any time.

It's important to remember that intrusive thoughts do not define us. They are simply products of our mind's habitual thinking patterns. Everyone experiences them at some point, and they are not necessarily an indication of our true desires or beliefs. In fact, trying to suppress them often strengthens their presence in our minds. This is where mindfulness comes into play. Through mindfulness, we can acknowledge these thoughts and then choose to release them without getting caught in their grip.

Mindfulness offers us a fresh approach to managing intrusive thoughts. Instead of letting these thoughts consume us, mindfulness teaches us to observe them as they arise, without judgment or attachment. With practice, we can learn to send these thoughts away, allowing them to pass as easily as they came. This process of letting go requires us to be present, to acknowledge the thought, and then choose not to engage with it. In this chapter, we will explore how we can use mindfulness to specifically release unwelcome thoughts from our minds, providing a step-by-step guide to gradually creating space for peace and calm.

The Role of Mindfulness in Dealing with Intrusive Thoughts

Mindfulness teaches us to be present with our experiences, including our thoughts, without judgment or attachment. This approach is crucial when dealing with intrusive thoughts because it helps us stop identifying with them. Rather than labeling ourselves as "someone who worries too much" or "someone who can't control their thoughts," mindfulness encourages us to observe our thoughts without attaching meaning or labels.

One of the most powerful aspects of mindfulness is its ability to help us create space between ourselves and our thoughts. Rather than becoming entangled in a thought, mindfulness allows us to observe it from a distance. This creates a sense of detachment, which reduces the emotional intensity of the thought. The more we practice this skill, the less power these intrusive thoughts will have over our mental state.

Sending Thoughts Out of Our Minds: A Step-by-Step Approach

The practice of sending intrusive thoughts out of our minds involves several mindful steps. It's about creating a conscious decision to not engage with the thought and choosing to let it pass by. Below is a step-by-step guide to help you learn how to send unwelcome thoughts out of your mind and regain a sense of control over your mental landscape.

1. Acknowledge the Thought

The first step in sending a thought away is to simply notice it. When an intrusive thought arises, acknowledge it without judgment. This may sound counterintuitive—after all, why would we want to acknowledge something that feels disruptive? But the key here is to recognize the thought without becoming emotionally invested in it.

For example, if the thought is about a mistake you made that day, you might say to yourself, "Ah, there's that thought again about my mistake." You are neither agreeing nor disagreeing with the thought; you are simply noticing its presence. By acknowledging the thought, you give yourself permission to observe it without getting caught up in it.

2. Label the Thought (Optional)

After acknowledging the thought, you may find it helpful to label it. This is an optional step, but it can help create further distance between yourself and the thought. Labeling can help you recognize that this thought is just one of many that will come and go throughout the day. It's not a reflection of who you are or what you believe.

For instance, if your intrusive thought is centered around fear of failure, you could label it as "fear" or "worry." If it's related to a past event that you regret, you might label it "regret." The label helps to reduce the intensity of the thought because it reframes it as a transient mental event, not a defining aspect of your identity.

In many cases, simply labeling the thought as "an intrusive thought" is enough to help regain control over it.

3. Visualize the Thought Leaving

Once you've acknowledged and labeled the thought, the next step is to visualize sending it out of your mind. Visualization is a powerful tool in mindfulness, and it can help you release thoughts in a physical and tangible way. The idea is to imagine the thought leaving your mental space in a manner that feels natural and easy.

One method is to imagine the thought as a balloon you release into the sky. Visualize it gradually drifting away, getting smaller and smaller as it moves further from you. Alternatively, you could picture the thought as a leaf floating down a stream, gently carried away by the current. Each time you see the thought moving away, you reinforce the notion that it is no longer relevant or important in this moment.

The key here is not to force the thought out but to simply give it permission to leave. The act of visualizing the thought leaving helps to reduce the emotional charge attached to it, allowing you to release it without feeling overwhelmed.

4. Return to the Present Moment

After visualizing the thought leaving, gently bring your attention back to the present moment. Focus on what is happening right now—your breath, the sensations in your body, the sounds around you. This serves to anchor you in the present, away from the intrusive thought. By focusing on the present moment, you remind yourself that the past or future, represented by the intrusive thought, no longer holds your attention.

You might find it helpful to take a few deep breaths to ground yourself further. With each inhale and exhale, remind yourself that you are in control of where you place your focus. As you continue to breathe, let the thought fade further into the background of your awareness.

5. Repeat the Process

Intrusive thoughts can be persistent, and they may return even after you've sent them away. When this happens, simply repeat the process. Each time the thought arises, acknowledge it, label it, and visualize it leaving your mind. The more you practice this process, the easier it becomes to release the thought.

It's important to be patient with yourself during this process. Some thoughts may take longer to dissipate than others, and that's okay. The goal isn't to suppress the thought or force it away, but to practice letting go of the attachment to it. With time, you'll find that these thoughts become less frequent and less disruptive.

6. Shift Focus to Something Positive

Once you've successfully sent the intrusive thought away, consider shifting your focus to something more positive or constructive. This could be an activity, a positive affirmation, or something that brings you joy or peace. The idea is to fill the mental space that was once occupied by the intrusive thought with something that enhances your well-being.

For example, you might shift your attention to something simple, like the feeling of your feet on the ground or the warmth of the sun on your face. Or, if you're dealing with a particularly challenging thought, you could repeat an affirmation such as, "I am in control of my mind," or "This thought does not define me."

Another option is to simply think about or visualize something unrelated to the intrusive thought that make you happy or brings you joy.

This shift in focus not only helps to replace the thought with something more positive, but it also reinforces your ability to manage your mental state with intention.

Releasing Intrusive Thoughts

Over time, as you continue to practice these mindfulness techniques, you'll notice that intrusive thoughts will become less overwhelming. The more you practice sending thoughts out, the less they will take hold of your attention. Mindfulness allows you to become more aware of your mental habits and create a sense of mental space that is not dominated by unwanted thoughts.

While intrusive thoughts may never fully disappear, mindfulness gives you the tools to manage them with greater ease. Rather than being overwhelmed by these thoughts, you can take an active role in deciding how to engage with them—or not. You can choose to send them away and return to a state of calm and presence, confident in your ability to manage your mind.

Creating Space for Peace and Clarity

Intrusive thoughts are a natural part of the human experience, but they don't have to control us. Through mindfulness, we can acknowledge these thoughts without attaching meaning to them, visualize them leaving our minds, and return our focus to the present moment. With practice, we can reduce the power of these thoughts and create more space for peace and clarity. By sending intrusive thoughts out, we gain greater control over our mental landscape, allowing us to move forward with a clearer, more constructive mindset.

CHAPTER 21: SETTING BOUNDARIES PROTECTING YOUR ENERGY AND MENTAL HEALTH

Setting boundaries is a crucial aspect of maintaining mental and emotional well-being. Boundaries define the space between you and others, ensuring that you are able to preserve your energy, time, and emotional resources. By being clear about what is acceptable and what is not, you create a framework within which you can interact with others in a healthy, balanced way.

Mindfulness offers a powerful tool in helping us understand, communicate, and maintain these boundaries. It provides us with the awareness to recognize our limits, the insight to honor those limits, and the ability to communicate them clearly and respectfully. This chapter will explore how mindfulness supports the establishment of boundaries, how it helps protect our emotional energy, and how it contributes to healthier, more balanced relationships.

Understanding Boundaries: The Foundation of Well-being

At the core of boundary-setting is the ability to define where your emotional and psychological space begins and ends. Boundaries are not about building walls between you and others; they are about knowing where you stop and another person begins. A boundary is essentially a clear line of respect for yourself and others. It ensures that your needs are met without compromising your well-being or sacrificing your emotional health.

Boundaries exist on multiple levels—physical, emotional, mental, and social—and are often influenced by your values, experiences, and beliefs. They are dynamic and can change over time, depending on the situation and context. For instance, your emotional boundaries may be more flexible with a close friend than with someone you have just met. Similarly, your physical boundaries may shift based on your comfort level or your relationship with a person.

When boundaries are not established or respected, emotional and mental strain can occur. Without boundaries, you may find yourself overextended, exhausted, or resentful. Conversely, healthy boundaries create a sense of security, allowing you to preserve your energy, maintain self-respect, and engage in relationships that feel nourishing rather than draining.

Mindfulness and the Recognition of Personal Limits

Mindfulness is the practice of being fully present in each moment, observing thoughts, feelings, and physical sensations without judgment. When it comes to setting boundaries, mindfulness helps you become more attuned to your own needs, limits, and emotional states. Through mindfulness, you can begin to recognize when you are reaching your limits—whether it's mentally, emotionally, or physically—and take appropriate action to honor those limits.

One of the core aspects of mindfulness is self-awareness. By cultivating a practice of mindfulness, you become more adept at noticing how situations, people, and experiences affect your mood, energy, and mental state. You begin to observe your reactions rather than merely reacting automatically. For example, when you feel your energy draining during a conversation or when your stress levels rise in a particular situation, mindfulness allows you to step back and recognize what is happening before you respond. This recognition is the first step in understanding your boundaries and acting in alignment with them.

Often, we push ourselves past our limits because we are not aware of the subtle signs that tell us we need rest, space, or a break. Through mindfulness, you can learn to recognize these signs early and make choices that protect your emotional and physical well-being.

Honoring Your Boundaries

Once you have developed the awareness of your personal limits, the next step is to honor them. Honoring your boundaries means acknowledging that you have the right to protect your energy and prioritize your well-being. This is not an act of selfishness but an essential practice of self-care. When you fail to honor your boundaries, you may find yourself drained, resentful, or overwhelmed.

Mindfulness supports this practice by helping you stay present with your emotions and needs. By regularly checking in with yourself—whether through deep breathing, reflection, or self-inquiry—you can gauge when a boundary needs to be set or reinforced. For example, when you are feeling mentally fatigued or emotionally depleted, mindfulness gives you the space to pause and decide whether you are in a position to continue engaging in a certain activity or interaction.

Honoring your boundaries requires strength and consistency. It may be difficult at times, especially when others' needs conflict with your own. However, mindfulness allows you to act in a way that is true to yourself, rather than succumbing to external pressures or internalized beliefs about what is expected of you. By maintaining mindfulness in these moments, you can say "no" or request a change without guilt or anxiety. When you honor your boundaries, you create space for healthier interactions and a greater sense of self-respect.

Communicating Boundaries Clearly and Respectfully

Mindfulness also plays a key role in communicating boundaries. In many cases, the challenge isn't recognizing your limits but expressing them to others in a way that is clear, respectful, and considerate. Whether in personal relationships, at work, or in social settings, being able to communicate your boundaries is essential for maintaining them.

Mindful communication encourages us to express ourselves honestly while remaining calm and composed. It involves being aware of how our words, tone, and body language can influence the conversation. By practicing mindful listening and speaking, we can approach these discussions with clarity and compassion.

For example, when someone asks for more of your time than you are able to give, a mindful response might be, "I value our time together, but right now I need to focus on my own responsibilities. Can we set a time to reconnect later?" By speaking clearly and respectfully, you set a boundary without guilt or defensiveness.

Mindful communication also involves checking in with yourself before responding. When a request is made that pushes against your boundaries, mindfulness allows you to pause and reflect before you react. This moment of reflection provides an opportunity to evaluate how you feel about the request and to consider how you can respond in a way that maintains your boundaries while honoring the other person's needs.

Navigating Guilt and Resistance

One of the common obstacles to setting and maintaining boundaries is guilt. Many people feel guilty when they assert their needs or decline requests, especially when they worry about disappointing others. This feeling of guilt often arises from a deeply ingrained belief that we should always prioritize others' needs above our own.

Mindfulness can help address this guilt by fostering self-compassion. Through mindfulness, you can become more attuned to the underlying emotions driving your guilt and recognize that it doesn't have to dictate your actions. Rather than pushing through guilt or ignoring it, mindfulness allows you to acknowledge it, sit with it, and choose how to respond. You can gently remind yourself that your boundaries are not only beneficial for you but also contribute to healthier, more balanced relationships.

Another challenge is the resistance we may face from others when we assert our boundaries. People may not always understand or respect our limits, and this can create discomfort or tension. Mindfulness can help us navigate these moments with grace. By staying grounded in the present moment and focusing on our own needs, we are less likely to get caught up in defensive reactions or to be swayed by others' emotions. Mindfulness helps us recognize that we are allowed to prioritize our own well-being, regardless of how others may respond.

Boundaries in Different Contexts

Boundaries are not one-size-fits-all. They vary depending on the context of the relationship and the situation at hand. For example, the boundaries you set with a close friend might differ from those you set with a colleague or a family member. The mindfulness practice encourages you to assess each situation with care and determine what is necessary for your emotional and mental well-being.

Physical boundaries are often the easiest to define. These include personal space and comfort levels regarding touch or proximity. However, emotional and psychological boundaries can be more complex. These boundaries involve how much of your emotional energy you are willing to give, what kind of behavior you are willing to tolerate, and how much personal information you are comfortable sharing.

Through mindfulness, you can evaluate your needs in different contexts. You might reflect on a situation after the fact, asking yourself how you felt about the interactions and whether your boundaries were respected. Over time, this reflection allows you to refine and strengthen your understanding of what you need in various contexts and how to communicate those needs effectively.

The Role of Boundaries in Healthy Relationships

At the heart of every healthy relationship is mutual respect for boundaries. When both parties in a relationship honor each other's limits, the relationship becomes more balanced, fulfilling, and harmonious. Boundaries foster respect, trust, and understanding. They allow each person to feel seen, heard, and valued.

Mindfulness can help you recognize when your boundaries are being respected and when they are being compromised. It helps you stay attuned to your emotional state, so you can gauge whether you feel comfortable or unsafe in a particular interaction. If you feel that your boundaries are being crossed, mindfulness gives you the clarity to address the situation directly and without fear.

Healthy relationships are based on mutual understanding and compromise, but they also require individuals to protect their own well-being. When both individuals in a relationship practice mindfulness and honor each other's boundaries, the relationship can thrive.

Promoting Wellbeing Through Boundary-Setting

Setting boundaries is an essential aspect of protecting your emotional and mental health. Mindfulness supports the process of recognizing, honoring, and communicating boundaries with clarity and compassion. By cultivating mindfulness, you become more attuned to your own needs and more capable of maintaining a balance in your relationships. This practice allows you to engage with others in a way that nurtures both your well-being and the well-being of those around you.

In doing so, you create space for healthier, more respectful interactions and cultivate a sense of peace and fulfillment in your life.

Through mindfulness, you learn to create and maintain boundaries that protect your energy and preserve your mental and emotional health, while fostering deeper, more meaningful connections with others. The ability to assert and honor your boundaries is not only an act of self-care but also an act of self-respect, allowing you to live in a way that is aligned with your values and needs.

CHAPTER 22: THE IMPORTANCE OF BALANCE

Balance is often described as a delicate equilibrium, something we strive for but rarely achieve permanently. It can seem like an ideal to be pursued but never fully attained. In reality, balance is not a static destination but a dynamic, ongoing process. It's about learning to adjust, adapt, and be aware of when we need to shift our focus, recalibrate our actions, or re-prioritize. Achieving balance is an art—one that requires constant awareness and a gentle, intentional approach. When it comes to living mindfully, balance becomes a powerful guiding principle that helps us manage the complexities of daily life, make thoughtful choices, and respond to challenges with clarity.

Mindfulness serves as the foundation for this balanced way of living. It teaches us that true balance is not about having everything perfectly in place, but rather about having the awareness to know when we're drifting off course. In the absence of mindfulness, it's easy to become overwhelmed by the demands of life, losing sight of what truly matters or spreading ourselves too thin. With mindfulness, we gain the clarity to make decisions that lead to a more harmonious, grounded existence.

The Quest for Balance

The concept of balance can sometimes feel elusive. We're often told that in order to live well, we must balance multiple areas of our lives—work, relationships, personal goals, and so on. But what does true balance mean? Is it about having equal attention or time for each area, or is it about giving each area the attention it truly needs in the moment?

This question is at the heart of the mindful approach to balance. Mindfulness helps answer this question by shifting our perspective from a rigid, one-size-fits-all view of balance to a more fluid, adaptive approach. Through mindfulness, we learn to approach balance not as something we must force or control, but as a practice of awareness and adaptation.

We often believe that balance requires equal distribution of time and energy across all areas of our lives. But mindfulness shows us that balance is more nuanced. It's about being fully present in each moment and responding thoughtfully to what life presents. By paying attention to our internal states, our actions, and our relationships, we start to recognize where we're leaning too far toward one thing or neglecting another. Mindfulness offers the clarity we need to restore harmony without forcing perfection.

When we live mindfully, we are not overwhelmed by the need to keep all aspects of life in perfect proportion. Rather, we become attuned to the natural ebb and flow of our daily rhythms. Some days may require more focus on work, while other days call for more attention to our relationships or personal goals. The key is awareness—the ability to recognize what needs our attention in the moment and make choices accordingly.

Living with Awareness of Priorities

At the core of achieving balance is the act of prioritization. We cannot do everything all at once, and trying to do so often leads to stress, exhaustion, and a sense of imbalance. Mindfulness, in this case, helps us become more attuned to our priorities and ensures we're focused on what matters most. When we're mindful, we become more attuned to our inner sense of what is important, what needs attention, and what can be set aside for a later time.

This mindful awareness helps us distinguish between what's urgent and what's important. We often confuse the two, reacting to every email, message, or task as though it's an urgent priority. Mindfulness teaches us the art of discernment, allowing us to respond intentionally, rather than react impulsively.

In our work lives, mindfulness helps us tune into the bigger picture. We can separate the essential from the non-essential, guiding us to focus on tasks that align with our long-term goals and values. This clarity creates balance in our work life, as we're not swept away by the constant pressure to do more, faster, or better. Instead, we operate from a place of purpose, knowing that we are focusing our energy on what matters most. With mindfulness, we see tasks for what they are, and rather than becoming stressed by the sheer volume of things we must accomplish, we address each one with intentional focus, maintaining balance even in the busiest of times.

Similarly, mindfulness helps us become more present in our relationships. By focusing on the needs and dynamics of our relationships, we're able to engage more meaningfully with those around us. Whether we're spending time with family, friends, or coworkers, mindfulness ensures we bring our full attention to the interaction, cultivating deeper connection and understanding. When we are mindful in our relationships, we avoid distractions and create space for meaningful exchanges that nourish and strengthen our connections.

Adapting to Change with Balance

Balance does not mean rigidity. It doesn't mean that everything must stay the same, or that we must maintain a fixed routine at all times. In fact, balance requires flexibility. It's about learning to adjust and adapt when life shifts unexpectedly.

Mindfulness supports this process by teaching us to stay grounded even as circumstances change. Life is inherently unpredictable, and our priorities, responsibilities, and circumstances can shift at any moment. Mindfulness helps us remain centered in these shifts, allowing us to adjust our focus when needed without becoming overwhelmed or reactive.

For example, if a personal issue arises that demands more of our attention, mindfulness enables us to be aware of this shift in energy and respond accordingly. We might need to focus more on our relationships or emotional well-being for a time, while reducing our attention on work or other commitments. Alternatively, if a new project arises at work, mindfulness allows us to allocate the necessary attention to that project while still staying grounded in other aspects of our life.

Through mindfulness, we learn that balance is dynamic and fluid, not something that can be rigidly controlled. In some moments, balance might look like investing more time in professional pursuits; in others, it may mean stepping back to nurture personal relationships or goals. Mindfulness allows us to make these adjustments with awareness, so that no aspect of our life is neglected or overburdened. The practice of balance is about recognizing that our needs and priorities shift, and responding to those shifts in ways that support our overall well-being.

The Practice of Balance in Everyday Life

Balance is not achieved in grand gestures, but in small, everyday actions and decisions. Each time we decide how to spend our energy, time, and attention, we are practicing balance. Every conversation, every task, every choice offers an opportunity to practice mindfulness and make decisions that reflect our values and priorities.

In our daily interactions, mindfulness helps us stay present with the people around us, creating a sense of equilibrium between our own needs and the needs of others. We learn to listen attentively, to respond thoughtfully, and to engage in relationships without losing ourselves in the process. When we are mindful, we avoid the tendency to rush through conversations, and instead, we approach each exchange with the full presence of mind. This presence enhances our relationships, making them more fulfilling and genuine.

In our work, mindfulness encourages us to focus on one task at a time, minimizing distractions and ensuring that we give each task the appropriate amount of focus and energy. Often, our desire to multitask leads to a sense of imbalance, as we attempt to juggle many things at once. Mindfulness shows us that by focusing fully on one task, we can actually accomplish more and with greater ease. Each task is given the space it needs to be done well, without unnecessary pressure or haste.

This balance extends to our physical space as well. When we practice mindfulness in our environment, we are more aware of the physical and mental clutter that can accumulate over time. We become mindful of the energy we expend in maintaining our space, which, in turn, creates a sense of peace and order. Intentionally creating a harmonious environment supports our overall sense of well-being, as our surroundings are often a reflection of our inner state.

When we are balanced in our surroundings, we find that the outside world reflects our inner harmony. Our workspace, home, and personal space become extensions of our internal balance. Mindfulness helps us cultivate an environment that supports focus, calm, and clarity, contributing to a greater sense of balance in our lives.

Balance as Part of an Interconnected System

One of the key aspects of mindfulness and balance is understanding that no area of life operates in isolation. Work, relationships, personal goals, and our internal well-being are all interconnected. When one area is out of balance, it can affect the others.

Mindfulness helps us see these connections clearly. If we're spending too much time focused on work, for example, we may start to feel disconnected from our relationships. Similarly, if we neglect our emotional health or well-being, it may impact our ability to engage fully in our work or relationships. Mindfulness helps us understand that true balance is not about isolating each area of life but about maintaining a sense of flow between them. Each area supports the others, and balance is achieved when we can move between these different aspects of our lives in a way that feels harmonious.

By practicing mindfulness, we gain the awareness necessary to recognize when something feels off-balance, whether it's our time, energy, or emotions. We become better at adjusting, allowing the different aspects of our lives to coexist and support one another in a fluid, organic way. This interconnectedness is vital in maintaining balance. Each part of our life is a thread in the larger tapestry, and mindfulness allows us to ensure that all threads are nurtured and maintained with care.

Mindfulness as a Continuous Practice

Balance is not a one-time achievement, but an ongoing practice. As we go through life, circumstances change, our priorities shift, and new challenges arise. Mindfulness helps us stay in touch with these shifts and remain responsive to our needs.

There will be times when we feel pulled in many directions, or when one area of life demands more attention than others. In these moments, mindfulness allows us to stay grounded and present, knowing that we can adjust when needed and return to a sense of balance as things settle. Mindfulness isn't about maintaining a perfect state of equilibrium but about maintaining awareness of what's needed in each moment and adjusting accordingly.

In essence, mindfulness helps us navigate the ever-shifting landscape of our lives with grace and clarity. By cultivating an awareness of where our attention is most needed, we can make more intentional choices that support a balanced, harmonious existence. Through mindfulness, we come to understand that balance isn't about strict rules or equal divisions of time and energy, but about the ongoing, conscious effort to live with purpose, awareness, and presence in all that we do.

Balance In Our Daily Lives

Balance is something we can practice every day, in every moment, through every decision we make. It's not about achieving perfection, but about creating harmony and alignment in our lives. Mindfulness gives us the tools to approach this practice with awareness, compassion, and clarity. Through mindfulness, we learn that balance is not something to be rigidly achieved, but something to be continuously cultivated with every conscious choice we make.

By integrating mindfulness into our daily lives, we become better equipped to live with intention, navigating the many demands and challenges with clarity and purpose. Balance is not a destination, but a journey—one that unfolds with each mindful step we take. With this awareness, we can live more fully and with greater intention, creating a life that feels both meaningful and harmonious.

CHAPTER 23: MINDFULNESS AND CREATIVE FREEDOM

Creativity is a free-flowing, dynamic force that thrives when we step aside from rigid expectations and allow ourselves to simply be in the moment. It is not something we create through effort or control, but something that emerges naturally when we release ourselves from preconceived outcomes and judgments. Creativity is the art of being open to what arises in the present moment—where ideas, emotions, and expressions can flow freely, without resistance.

At its core, creativity is an act of freedom. It is a state where we are unrestricted by limitations or fixed outcomes, where our thoughts and actions move freely within the space we create. It is not bound by structure or expectation, but rather exists in the fluidity between form and formlessness. This kind of creative freedom exists not in an absence of structure, but in the harmony between openness and intention, spontaneity and direction. The creative process is, at its essence, about being present—letting go of control and simply allowing the experience to unfold.

Mindfulness is the doorway through which we enter this creative freedom. It allows us to tap into the fluidity of creativity by rooting us in the present moment, where we can engage with the world and our inner landscapes without interference. When we are mindful, we are not distracted by self-judgment or outside pressures. We are fully immersed in the process of creation, free from the fear of failure or the need to achieve perfection. In this state, creativity flows effortlessly. We can connect deeply with the act of creating, allowing inspiration to arise without resistance.

The creative process is never linear. It is not a step-by-step procedure but a constant ebb and flow. It is a dance between openness and focus, between structure and spontaneity. And just as the tides of the ocean shift and change with every moment, so too does the creative flow. To participate fully in this flow requires mindfulness—the ability to be present with whatever arises and to respond with flexibility and ease.

The Art of Letting Go

Creativity does not thrive under pressure or in the presence of judgment. When we hold ourselves to high standards or expect perfection from the outset, we constrict the natural flow of inspiration. Mindfulness provides a release from this tension. It teaches us to be open and to embrace uncertainty. When we let go of the need to control the outcome of our creative work, we free ourselves to explore, to experiment, and to discover what we might not have known was even possible. We give ourselves permission to create freely, without fear of imperfection, knowing that each step is part of the journey and that every mistake is a part of the creative process itself.

Letting go of expectations is a key principle of mindfulness, and this same principle applies directly to creativity. The less we cling to preconceived notions of how something "should" turn out, the more space we create for fresh ideas to emerge. In this way, mindfulness doesn't just help clear mental clutter; it actively fosters a fertile environment for creative thought to arise.

This freedom, however, does not mean abandoning all structure. It means allowing the structure to emerge naturally as we go along. Instead of rigidly forcing a plan into existence, we let the work evolve, adapting to the flow of ideas as they come. This fluidity is what allows creativity to be such a powerful force—it is not bound by limitations, but shaped by an openness to possibility.

Fluidity and Flexibility

Creativity is inherently fluid. It cannot be contained by formulas or fixed methods. It moves and shifts with every new insight, every new connection, and every new direction. The mind that is fully present can tap into this fluidity, moving effortlessly from one thought to another, one idea to the next. It is in this space of fluid thinking that the most original and innovative ideas often appear.

Mindfulness teaches us to approach creativity with this same fluidity. It encourages us to be present without forcing outcomes. In the practice of mindfulness, there is no rushing, no striving to arrive at a destination. Instead, there is a trust in the process, a belief that ideas will come and go, and that the creative flow will shift as needed. The act of creation becomes an open space where we are free to explore and experiment without concern for the end result.

In a fluid state of mind, we can pivot from one creative direction to another without hesitation, moving with the changes rather than resisting them. This fluidity gives us the freedom to experiment, to try new things, to explore without limitation. Creativity, in its purest form, cannot be forced; it must be nurtured in a space of openness and flexibility.

Freedom Through Presence

The creative process flourishes in the absence of distraction. To be truly creative, we must immerse ourselves fully in the present moment. Mindfulness allows us to do this. By focusing our attention on the here and now, we remove distractions and make space for creativity to emerge. When we are present, we are not clouded by concerns about the future or past; we are fully engaged with the current moment and what it has to offer.

This presence is crucial for creative freedom. It is only when we are fully present that we can truly engage with the process of creation. Mindfulness teaches us to be present with our ideas, with the materials we are working with, and with the act of creating itself. When we practice being in the moment, we can connect more deeply with our creativity, allowing it to flow freely and without inhibition.

Being present in the moment also allows us to see things with fresh eyes. We can approach our work without preconceived notions, without the filter of expectations. This is where true innovation happens—when we engage with our creative work as if it is new, as if we have never seen it before, and when we are open to whatever arises.

Creativity in Play

Mindfulness encourages us to bring a sense of play into our creative process. It invites us to approach our work with curiosity and openness, to try new things without fear of failure. In this playful state, we are free to explore, to test ideas, and to experiment with abandon. We are not concerned with making mistakes because we understand that mistakes are part of the process. Instead of seeing setbacks as failures, we view them as opportunities to learn, grow, and shift direction.

The playful nature of creativity is enhanced when we are not bogged down by self-doubt or judgment. Mindfulness helps us detach from these negative thought patterns, allowing us to be more playful, more experimental, and more open to new ideas. We learn to approach our creative work with a sense of wonder, not concern.

Creativity as an Ongoing Journey

Creativity is not a destination—it is an ongoing process, one that is ever-changing and evolving. As we engage with our creative work, we enter into a continuous dialogue with our ideas, our thoughts, and our emotions. Mindfulness supports this process by encouraging us to stay present, to remain engaged with whatever arises, and to trust the journey of creation.

Each moment of the creative process brings something new. There are no fixed outcomes, no final answers. Instead, there is a constant unfolding, a continual expansion of ideas and insights. This journey is never static. It is fluid, dynamic, and ever-shifting. And through mindfulness, we learn to embrace this fluidity, to trust that the creative process will unfold in its own time and in its own way.

The key to creative freedom is not in controlling the process, but in allowing it to flow naturally. Mindfulness teaches us to let go of the need to direct every step and instead to be present with each phase of the journey. We learn to adapt, to pivot, and to flow with the changes as they come. In doing so, we create the conditions in which our creativity can truly thrive.

The Aliveness of Creative Freedom

Creative freedom is not merely about producing something new; it is about the aliveness of the process itself. It is about being fully immersed in the act of creating, without distraction or inhibition. Mindfulness connects us to this aliveness by keeping us present and engaged with the creative act. When we are present, we are not just creating in the sense of producing something; we are experiencing the act of creation itself. The act of making becomes an expression of who we are in that moment, fully alive and engaged with the process.

Through mindfulness, we create an open space for creativity to flow freely, for ideas to come and go, and for innovation to emerge. We let go of the need to control, and instead embrace the freedom of creation in all its unpredictability. This freedom is what makes creativity so powerful—it is the ability to explore, experiment, and express ourselves without boundaries or limitations.

CHAPTER 24: FINDING MEANING IN SMALL MOMENTS

It can be easy to overlook the small moments that make up the fabric of our daily experience. We are conditioned to think that meaning and fulfillment lie in major achievements or in moments that stand out as exceptional. However, the true richness of life is found not in grand events but in the ordinary moments we often pass by without a second thought.

Mindfulness, the practice of being fully present and aware in the current moment, opens the door to these small but meaningful experiences. Through mindfulness, we become aware of the beauty and depth that can be found in what might seem like mundane activities. The ability to connect deeply with small moments is not only a source of joy but also a means of cultivating meaning in our lives, helping us live more fully and with greater appreciation for the present.

The Power of Small Moments

Most of our days are filled with ordinary tasks: making coffee, washing dishes, walking to the store, having brief conversations, or simply sitting still for a few moments. In our culture, these small moments are often dismissed as unimportant compared to bigger events. However, meaning is often hidden in plain sight, in the simplicity of these everyday moments. When we practice mindfulness, we shift our attention from the next big thing to the richness of the present moment.

Meaning isn't always found in the extraordinary. It is embedded in the quiet, the small, and the subtle. We might believe that true fulfillment comes from reaching certain milestones or achieving particular goals, but what happens when we learn to slow down and pay attention to what is right in front of us? The small moments are where life unfolds, and by being present with them, we can tap into their inherent richness.

Imagine a moment of stillness, like the quiet before dawn. It's easy to dismiss, but when we are mindful of it, we realize how it offers a sense of calm, a break from the noise that may otherwise fill our lives. Similarly, the simple act of sitting down to enjoy a meal, without distraction or hurry, can become a moment of mindfulness, allowing us to savor the flavors, the textures, and the sensation of nourishment.

Mindfulness: The Key to Finding Meaning

At its core, mindfulness is the practice of bringing our full attention to the present moment. It invites us to observe our thoughts, feelings, and experiences without judgment, allowing us to fully experience the world as it is. This practice is essential in helping us uncover meaning in small moments. When we slow down and engage fully with the present, we are able to experience the depth of each moment, which may otherwise be overlooked.

Mindfulness shifts our perspective, helping us realize that there is meaning to be found in every aspect of life. The feeling of the sun on our skin, the sound of a bird calling in the distance, the taste of a cup of tea—each of these moments, when experienced with mindfulness, has the potential to be deeply fulfilling. Meaning, then, does not need to be a complex or elusive concept; it exists within the small, simple experiences we encounter every day.

Through mindfulness, we develop the ability to be fully present in the moment, which helps us feel more connected to ourselves and the world around us. We notice things that we might have missed before—the intricate patterns of leaves on a tree, the way light shifts throughout the day, the subtleties in someone's voice during a conversation. These small moments, once we become mindful of them, begin to take on a deeper significance.

Slowing Down to Experience the Present

In order to find meaning in the small moments, it is essential that we slow down. Much of our daily lives are rushed, as we move from one task to the next with little thought to what is happening in the present. This speed often prevents us from fully appreciating what is in front of us. By rushing through life, we bypass the opportunity to experience the richness of the present moment.

Mindfulness teaches us to slow down, to step out of the cycle of constant doing, and to be fully present. This doesn't mean that we stop doing things or slow down our productivity—it means that we stop and take notice of what we are doing and how we are feeling in the moment. We engage in the task at hand with complete awareness, allowing us to experience the process rather than focusing solely on the outcome.

Slowing down allows us to notice the subtleties that make each moment unique. For example, when walking, we may pay attention to how our feet feel as they meet the ground, the rhythm of our breathing, or the changing scenery around us. These simple acts can become moments of meaning when we approach them with mindfulness. Instead of rushing from one place to the next, we give ourselves the gift of being fully present, and in doing so, we create space for meaning to emerge.

Finding Joy in the Everyday

When we begin to see the beauty in small moments, we also begin to find joy in the simple, everyday tasks. Mindfulness helps us shift our focus away from the idea that joy can only be found in big events, special occasions, or achievements. Instead, we realize that joy is available to us at any moment, simply by being present and appreciating what is happening right now.

Take, for instance, the act of drinking a cup of tea. When done mindfully, this simple activity becomes an opportunity to appreciate the warmth of the cup, the fragrance of the tea, and the act of nourishing our body. This experience, when lived fully in the moment, brings a sense of peace and contentment. It's a reminder that joy can be found in the quiet, the subtle, and the small.

Similarly, the practice of mindful eating can turn every meal into a moment of joy and appreciation. Instead of eating while distracted or hurried, we take the time to savor each bite, noticing the texture, the flavors, and the sensations that come with it. This act of mindful eating not only enhances our enjoyment but also helps us develop a deeper relationship with food, our body, and the nourishment we receive.

By turning our attention to the small moments, we open ourselves to a constant stream of opportunities for joy and fulfillment. These moments may seem insignificant on their own, but when added up, they form the foundation of a meaningful life.

Reflection: Deepening Our Connection to the Present Moment

Mindfulness is not just about being present in the moment—it is also about reflection. Reflection helps us understand the significance of the moments we experience, allowing us to see how they contribute to our overall sense of meaning. After engaging with a small moment mindfully, reflection helps us integrate the experience and explore what it means for us.

For example, after taking a mindful walk in nature, we might reflect on how we felt during the walk—the sense of peace, the stillness, the beauty around us. By reflecting on these feelings, we deepen our connection to the experience and notice how it impacted our mood or perspective. We begin to understand how these small moments shape our well-being, and we learn to appreciate them more fully.

Reflection also helps us connect the present moment to our larger life goals, values, and desires. By reflecting on our experiences, we gain insight into what truly matters to us, what brings us peace, and what helps us feel fulfilled. This process can help guide our actions, decisions, and relationships, allowing us to live more intentionally.

The Art of Mindful Appreciation

Another important aspect of finding meaning in small moments is the practice of appreciation. When we are mindful, we become more aware of what is happening around us, and we begin to recognize the beauty and value in even the simplest experiences. Appreciation shifts our focus from what is lacking to what is already present, helping us cultivate a deeper sense of gratitude and contentment.

Mindful appreciation can take many forms. It might be as simple as appreciating the sound of birds chirping in the morning or the feeling of warmth from the sun on our skin. It might be noticing the way light shifts throughout the day or taking pleasure in a shared moment with a friend. The practice of appreciation helps us stay grounded in the present moment, recognizing that meaning is found in the small, ordinary aspects of life.

The more we practice mindful appreciation, the more we begin to see that life is not about waiting for extraordinary moments to happen. It is about finding the extraordinary within the ordinary, recognizing the richness that already exists in our everyday experiences.

Living in the Present

Ultimately, meaning is not something we need to seek outside of ourselves. It is found right where we are, in the small moments that make up our day. Mindfulness teaches us to become fully engaged with the present moment, and in doing so, we discover that meaning is not a distant goal but something that unfolds in each passing second.

By slowing down, reflecting, appreciating, and engaging with life mindfully, we begin to uncover the depth of meaning that exists in every moment. The small moments are not filler in between bigger events; they are the events themselves. When we learn to appreciate and experience them fully, we create a life that is rich with meaning, joy, and fulfillment.

In this way, mindfulness helps us build a deeper connection to ourselves and the world around us. It teaches us that meaning is not something we need to search for—it is already here, in the small, quiet moments that make up our everyday lives. Through mindfulness, we can discover the richness of life in its simplest form, and in doing so, live a life that is truly meaningful.

CHAPTER 25: THE HEALING POWER OF NATURE

There is something inherently healing about nature. Its calm and simplicity have the power to restore our minds, nurture our bodies, and uplift our spirits. Whether it's the vastness of a mountain range, the quiet of a forest, or the serene beauty of a garden, nature has a way of bringing us back to ourselves. It serves as a reminder of the balance, order, and peace that exists in the world, offering us a chance to reconnect and heal in ways that other environments cannot.

The Connection Between Nature and Well-being

From the moment we step outside, nature has an immediate effect on us. It is a constant presence in our lives, whether we are aware of it or not. The outdoors, in all its various forms, invites us to slow down and become present with what is around us. By doing so, we often find a sense of calm that might be difficult to access in other settings. Nature offers an environment that encourages us to let go of the clutter of our minds and the distractions of our daily routines. In this way, it becomes a sanctuary—an oasis where we can relax, refresh, and restore.

Being in nature provides an opportunity to quiet the mind and find balance. When we are surrounded by trees, mountains, rivers, or even a simple patch of grass, we naturally become more aware of our surroundings. The sounds of birds, the rustling of leaves, or the flow of water can all serve as gentle reminders to be present. The act of simply observing nature allows us to take a step back, let go of distractions, and experience a moment of peace.

Mental and Emotional Healing

Nature's ability to heal is rooted in its ability to foster mindfulness. Mindfulness is the practice of being fully present and aware, without judgment or attachment. In nature, mindfulness can arise effortlessly. When we immerse ourselves in a natural environment, we are often drawn to focus on the details—whether it's the scent of fresh air, the texture of bark, or the movement of clouds. This heightened awareness naturally redirects our attention away from stress, worries, and mental noise.

The act of being in nature invites reflection and introspection, providing a space where we can release negative emotions. Stress, anxiety, and worry can often seem overwhelming, but nature offers us a place to reset. When we are able to focus on the beauty and stillness around us, we often find that our emotional state begins to shift. Negative emotions lose their grip, allowing us to experience relief and emotional clarity.

Nature also offers us a gentle reminder of the impermanence of life. As we witness the changing seasons, the cycles of life and death in plants and animals, we are reminded that everything is temporary. This perspective allows us to release attachments and judgments about our own lives, fostering greater emotional resilience. Nature teaches us that growth and change are inevitable parts of existence, and by embracing this truth, we can approach challenges with a sense of ease.

Physical Well-being

Spending time in nature isn't just beneficial for our mental and emotional health—it also supports our physical well-being. Engaging in outdoor activities, whether it's a walk through a park or sitting by a lakeside, brings a sense of calm to the body. Nature helps us release physical tension, lower our heart rates, and reduce feelings of stress.

Taking a nature walk is one of the simplest and most effective ways to integrate nature's healing power into our lives. The act of walking itself promotes circulation, eases joint stiffness, and improves muscle tone. But when we walk in nature, these physical benefits are magnified by the soothing influence of our surroundings. The sights and sounds of nature help us relax further, while the act of walking in a natural setting encourages a steady rhythm that allows our bodies to settle into a peaceful state.

The rhythm of walking can also serve as a form of moving meditation. As you walk along a trail, through a park, or even along the beach, you can allow your focus to shift away from the busyness of the world and into the present moment. Each step becomes a grounding experience, connecting you to the earth beneath your feet. You might notice the texture of the path, the sound of your footsteps, or the sensation of the wind against your skin. This focus on the act of walking brings mindfulness to the experience, helping to release tension and bring a sense of harmony to your body and mind.

Even the air itself can be healing. Clean, fresh air can bring a sense of vitality and energy. Breathing deeply during a nature walk allows us to fill our lungs with oxygen, refresh our body, and clear our mind. This simple act of breathing in nature's purity is one of the most effective ways to feel rejuvenated. In addition, the natural light, especially when walking outside during the day, helps regulate our circadian rhythms and improves our overall sense of well-being.

Nature also promotes restful sleep. The combination of physical movement, exposure to natural light, and time spent in a calming environment can improve our ability to sleep soundly at night. The restorative qualities of nature linger long after we leave it, influencing how we rest and recover.

Mindfulness in Nature

When we combine the act of spending time in nature with the practice of mindfulness, we deepen the healing potential of the experience. Nature becomes a powerful backdrop for cultivating awareness and presence. There are various ways to approach mindfulness in nature, but the underlying principle remains the same: to be fully present with whatever is happening in the moment, without distraction or judgment.

One of the simplest ways to practice mindfulness in nature is through focused observation. As we walk through a forest or sit in a garden, we can take the time to notice the details around us. What do we hear? What do we see? What do we smell? Focusing on these sensory details allows us to become more attuned to the environment and to the present moment. We begin to appreciate the subtleties of the world around us—the shifting patterns of light, the texture of the ground beneath our feet, or the rhythm of the wind.

Another form of mindfulness in nature is simply being still. In a world that often encourages constant movement, taking time to simply sit and observe can be transformative. Find a quiet spot in nature, close your eyes for a moment, and take in the sounds of the environment. This practice of sitting still and breathing deeply allows us to ground ourselves and reconnect with the earth. When we sit in nature, we open ourselves to its healing energy and its ability to calm the mind.

Eco-Mindfulness: Connecting with the Earth

Mindfulness in nature also has an ecological component, often referred to as eco-mindfulness. This practice invites us to become more aware of our relationship with the environment and to cultivate a sense of responsibility for its well-being. By practicing mindfulness in nature, we develop a deeper appreciation for the natural world and the interconnectedness of all living things.

When we engage with nature mindfully, we begin to recognize the fragility and beauty of our planet. This awareness encourages us to take care of our environment, not just for our own well-being, but for the well-being of future generations. Eco-mindfulness inspires actions that are aligned with the values of sustainability and environmental stewardship.

By being mindful of nature, we also acknowledge our place within it. We are part of the natural world, and when we treat it with care and respect, we are nurturing ourselves as well. Practicing eco-mindfulness may involve simple acts like reducing waste, planting trees, or supporting conservation efforts. But it also involves shifting our mindset to one of interconnectedness and respect for the environment.

Incorporating Nature into Daily Life

While taking long trips into nature can be deeply restorative, the benefits of nature can be integrated into everyday life. There are many simple ways to connect with the outdoors, even if you don't have access to vast natural spaces. Spending time in a local park, tending to a garden, or simply stepping outside for a few minutes each day can have a profound impact on your well-being.

When we make nature a regular part of our routine, we create an opportunity for daily healing. It doesn't require long hours or grand gestures—just moments of mindful presence in the natural world. These small acts of connection build over time, contributing to a greater sense of balance and tranquility. Taking a walk in the park or around your neighborhood every day can be a small yet powerful practice of connecting with nature and its healing power. The quiet moments during these walks can bring calm, clarity, and a sense of rejuvenation, all while improving your physical health.

The Power to Heal

Nature holds a quiet power to heal, refresh, and restore us. When we immerse ourselves in natural surroundings, we create space for mindfulness, reflection, and peace. The healing power of nature is both immediate and lasting, offering benefits for our mental, emotional, and physical health. By connecting with nature regularly and practicing mindfulness in these environments, we nurture our bodies, soothe our minds, and foster a deeper appreciation for the world around us. The healing power of nature is always available, waiting for us to step outside and embrace its simple, yet profound, gifts.

CHAPTER 26:
MINDFULNESS
AND SELF-CARE

Prioritizing Your Well-being

Taking care of yourself is one of the most important and rewarding commitments you can make. It's not only about indulgence or treating yourself as a reward for hard work, but about honoring your needs with the same care and attention you give to others. When you approach self-care through mindfulness, it becomes more than just an occasional act—it transforms into a regular practice that nurtures your mind, body, and spirit in a balanced and thoughtful way. Through mindfulness, you cultivate an awareness of your well-being that helps you meet the demands of daily life without sacrificing your peace, energy, or joy.

Mindfulness, in the context of self-care, is more than a prescriptive set of actions. It is a practice of deep listening—attuning yourself to your own needs, recognizing when you're out of balance, and responding in ways that restore harmony. In this chapter, we will explore how mindfulness can serve as a foundation for a rich and fulfilling self-care routine that goes beyond the surface and touches on the deeper, more subtle ways we can care for ourselves every day.

Cultivating Awareness of Your Needs

Mindfulness starts with awareness—being present with what's happening in the moment, both internally and externally. In the hustle and bustle of everyday life, it's easy to overlook our own needs. Whether we're caught up in our to-do lists, other people's expectations, or the pressures of work, we often forget to pause and check in with ourselves.

But when we practice mindfulness, we create space to tune into our thoughts, feelings, and physical sensations. We begin to notice when we feel overwhelmed, stressed, or fatigued, and we learn to interpret these signals without judgment. Instead of pushing through discomfort or ignoring subtle signs of burnout, mindfulness invites us to recognize these signals as important information about what we need at that moment.

This practice of noticing is foundational to self-care. It allows us to make choices that reflect what we truly require, whether that's rest, quiet, connection, or simply a change of scenery. Mindfulness allows us to respond in the way that best nurtures our well-being rather than reacting based on external pressures or unconscious habits.

Making Time for Yourself

One of the most significant ways mindfulness supports self-care is by helping us carve out time for ourselves in a way that feels authentic and nurturing. We live in a world where our time is constantly demanded by others, and many people feel that taking time for themselves is selfish or unproductive. However, mindfulness reminds us that making time for our own well-being is essential to our ability to show up fully in all areas of life.

Self-care is a necessary practice. Just as a plant needs regular watering and sunlight to thrive, we need regular moments to recharge, reflect, and reconnect with ourselves. Mindfulness encourages us to see this time not as something indulgent or frivolous, but as an investment in our long-term well-being. When we make time for ourselves, we ensure that we have the energy, mental clarity, and emotional resilience to meet the demands of our day.

Creating time for self-care through mindfulness may look different for each person. It might involve setting aside moments of quiet each day to sit in reflection or dedicating time each week to engage in a hobby or activity that brings you joy. Whether it's a few minutes of mindfulness practice or a longer period of rest, these moments allow you to reconnect with your inner self and restore your energy.

Responding to Your Body's Signals

Our bodies are often the first to communicate when we need self-care. Physical discomfort, tension, or fatigue can be signs that our bodies need attention, yet we often push through these sensations, hoping they will go away. Mindfulness helps us stay attuned to our bodies, recognizing these signals as invitations to slow down and check in with ourselves.

When we practice mindfulness, we learn to pay attention to the physical sensations that arise throughout the day. Whether it's noticing the tension in our shoulders, the tightness in our chest, or the tiredness in our eyes, mindfulness helps us tune into these sensations and take appropriate action. Sometimes, this means taking a break to stretch or breathe deeply. Other times, it could be acknowledging that we need rest or changing our physical posture to alleviate discomfort.

Through mindfulness, we shift from ignoring or bypassing our body's needs to responding with care and respect. This allows us to avoid physical strain, prevent burnout, and maintain a sense of vitality and well-being throughout the day. Mindful attention to the body becomes a powerful tool for supporting long-term health, improving energy levels, and preventing unnecessary stress or discomfort.

Mental and Emotional Care Through Mindfulness

While physical self-care is essential, mental and emotional care is just as important. Mindfulness plays a pivotal role in helping us maintain mental clarity and emotional resilience. In the fast-moving nature of life, we can easily become overwhelmed by our thoughts and emotions. Mindfulness encourages us to become observers of our mental and emotional states rather than becoming overwhelmed by them.

The practice of mindfulness allows us to become more aware of our thoughts and feelings without getting caught up in them. This means noticing when we're feeling stressed, anxious, or upset without immediately reacting. Instead, mindfulness encourages us to observe these emotions with curiosity, acknowledging them as valid but not necessarily permanent states.

By creating space between our emotional responses and actions, mindfulness allows us to make decisions that align with our true needs rather than reacting out of stress or frustration. It helps us release judgment about our emotions, allowing us to experience them fully without getting stuck in negative patterns. Through mindfulness, we learn to care for our mental and emotional well-being by creating a compassionate and non-judgmental space where we can process our feelings.

Mindfulness in Everyday Actions

Self-care doesn't have to be grand or extravagant—it can be built into the simple actions of our day. Mindfulness shows us how even the smallest moments can contribute to our well-being. Whether it's taking a mindful walk, or simply pausing for a deep breath in between tasks, mindfulness helps us bring a sense of awareness and presence to each action.

When we apply mindfulness to everyday activities, we cultivate a greater sense of peace and satisfaction. We stop rushing through tasks and instead embrace the experience of doing them. Washing dishes can become an act of mindfulness, as we focus on the feel of the warm water and the sensation of each dish in our hands. We can approach even the most mundane tasks with presence and care, turning them into moments of self-nurturance.

Mindfulness also helps us avoid the trap of overloading our

schedules. When we take time to check in with ourselves throughout the day, we recognize when we're pushing ourselves too hard or taking on more than we can handle. It allows us to prioritize what truly matters and let go of activities or commitments that drain our energy.

Letting Go of Overwhelm

When life feels overwhelming, mindfulness helps us find clarity. It gives us the tools to step back, observe the situation from a distance, and discern what is most important in that moment. Instead of getting swept away by a long list of tasks, mindfulness teaches us to approach each moment with a sense of calm and clarity.

By practicing mindfulness, we can break down tasks into smaller, more manageable pieces and focus on the present task at hand. Instead of worrying about everything we have to do, mindfulness invites us to focus on what we can do in this moment, allowing us to release the anxiety of trying to control everything. This mental clarity makes it easier to let go of overwhelm and prioritize our well-being.

Mindfulness also helps us recognize the limits of our own capacity. It encourages us to listen to our internal signals and step back when we need to rest. By respecting these boundaries, we protect ourselves from burnout and exhaustion, ensuring that we have the energy to continue showing up in meaningful ways.

Nurturing the Soul Through Presence

Mindfulness is about being fully present with ourselves and with our experiences. It's about being aware of the here and now, without rushing toward the future or dwelling in the past. When we practice mindfulness, we cultivate a deeper connection with our own essence. This connection is nourishing for our soul, offering us a sense of calm and contentment that is independent of external circumstances.

Being present in each moment allows us to experience life more fully and deeply. Whether we're enjoying a simple meal, having a conversation with a friend, or walking outside, mindfulness helps us savor the richness of each experience. This presence nurtures our sense of self-worth and reinforces our commitment to care for ourselves.

Mindfulness reminds us that we are worthy of care, attention, and respect. It helps us honor our unique needs and supports us in creating a life that is aligned with our values and desires.

Mindfulness and Self-Care

Self-care is a necessary and essential practice for maintaining our well-being. Through mindfulness, we learn to cultivate awareness of our needs, listen to our bodies, and make intentional choices that nurture our mental, emotional, and physical health. By weaving mindfulness into our daily lives, we turn self-care into a continuous practice that nurtures us in every moment, rather than something we reserve for special occasions.

Mindfulness supports us in responding to our own needs with clarity and compassion, allowing us to maintain balance, reduce stress, and approach life with a deeper sense of connection to ourselves. It helps us nurture not just our bodies, but our minds and emotions as well, creating a holistic and balanced approach to self-care.

Ultimately, mindfulness teaches us that taking care of ourselves can be an act of honoring our own value by maintaining our wellbeing. By making self-care a priority, we not only enhance our own lives but also become better equipped to contribute to the well-being of others. In practicing mindfulness, we create the space to live a life that is grounded in peace, health, and authentic self-care.

CHAPTER 27: MINDFULNESS AND SELF-REFLECTION

Self-reflection, when practiced with mindfulness, offers an enriching approach to understanding ourselves more deeply. While mindfulness encourages us to be fully present in the moment, self-reflection invites us to pause, look inward, and examine our thoughts, actions, and feelings. These practices allow us to gain deeper insight into our motivations, actions, and emotions. Mindfulness helps clear our minds, allowing self-reflection to become a tool for understanding and growth.

The Role of Mindfulness in Self-Reflection

At its core, mindfulness is about cultivating awareness of the present moment without judgment. This process involves noticing our thoughts, emotions, and physical sensations as they arise, allowing them to come and go naturally without being swept away by them. When we are mindful, we are less likely to become entangled in our thoughts or overwhelmed by emotions. We observe them as they are, without attaching labels or judgments.

Self-reflection, on the other hand, is the process of stepping back and reviewing our actions, thoughts, and feelings. It's about asking ourselves questions such as, "Why did I feel that way?" or "What motivated me to respond in that manner?" Through self-reflection, we attempt to make sense of our experiences, gain clarity about our behavior, and uncover deeper insights into our motivations.

When we integrate mindfulness into self-reflection, we create a calm, objective space where we can look at ourselves with kindness and curiosity. Mindfulness encourages us to engage with the process of reflection without criticism or the urge to "fix" ourselves immediately. Instead, it allows us to observe our experiences with patience, recognizing that growth and self-understanding take time. This is a critical distinction —mindfulness helps us reflect with greater awareness and compassion, which ultimately allows us to gain clarity and move forward with intention.

Observing Without Judgment

One of the primary challenges of self-reflection is our tendency to judge ourselves. It's easy to slip into negative thinking, whether we're criticizing past decisions, feeling guilty about certain actions, or regretting missed opportunities. This self-judgment, however, often obscures the process of meaningful reflection. When we judge ourselves harshly, we create resistance to seeing the truth. We may become defensive or closed off to understanding the full range of our experiences.

Mindfulness directly addresses this challenge by cultivating non-judgmental awareness. It encourages us to observe our thoughts and feelings without immediately labeling them as good or bad. Instead of thinking, "I shouldn't have acted like that," mindfulness allows us to notice the thought or emotion without attaching any judgment to it. By approaching our reflections without criticism, we remove the internal barriers that can prevent growth.

Self-reflection from a mindful perspective can become a tool for exploration rather than self-criticism. We begin to ask, "What can I learn from this experience?" instead of "Why did I mess up?" This shift in perspective can be transformative. It enables us to examine our experiences from a place of curiosity rather than shame or guilt. Without judgment, we gain access to deeper layers of understanding about ourselves, our behaviors, and our emotional responses.

Deepening Understanding of the Self Through Mindful Reflection

Self-reflection offers an opportunity to look at ourselves with fresh eyes. Our thoughts and feelings may be so familiar that we become desensitized to their influence. We might not even realize the underlying assumptions or patterns that guide our actions. Mindfulness provides the space to observe these patterns without being consumed by them.

The process of reflecting can help us identify recurring thought patterns and emotional responses. When we become aware of these tendencies, we can start to understand the "why" behind our behavior. Are we reacting to situations out of fear? Are we avoiding difficult emotions or memories? Are our actions driven by external pressures or societal expectations? Through mindfulness, we can observe these patterns without judgment, which is the first step in understanding them.

Mindfulness can help us avoid getting lost in the past or future while reflecting. Often, we reflect on past mistakes or missed opportunities, which may bring feelings of regret or frustration. Alternatively, we may dwell on future scenarios, worrying about what's to come. Mindfulness anchors us in the present, where we can reflect without being consumed by these thoughts. It allows us to examine our past or future experiences with a clearer, more balanced perspective, helping us move beyond regret and anxiety.

Clarity Through Mindful Awareness

Self-reflection without mindfulness can often feel overwhelming. We may try to understand a situation, but the mind's clutter of worries, judgments, and assumptions makes it difficult to see things clearly. Mindfulness helps cut through this mental fog by providing clarity.

When we practice mindfulness, we learn to quiet the noise in our minds and focus on what's happening in the present moment. This calm, focused awareness gives us a clearer lens through which to view our thoughts, emotions, and experiences. The clarity gained through mindfulness helps us engage in self-reflection more effectively. We are less likely to get lost in overthinking or rumination, and we are better able to see things for what they truly are.

This clarity can also help us gain perspective on difficult emotions. When we are caught in a strong emotional reaction, such as anger or sadness, it can be hard to think clearly. Mindfulness allows us to notice these emotions as they arise and experience them without becoming consumed by them. In turn, self-reflection becomes a more balanced process. Instead of reflecting from a place of emotional intensity, we can reflect from a place of calm, which gives us the space to process our feelings and understand their origins.

Cultivating Self-Compassion Through Reflection

Another powerful aspect of mindfulness is its ability to cultivate self-compassion. Mindful self-reflection encourages us to approach our past mistakes, regrets, or difficult emotions with kindness and understanding. Often, when we reflect on our shortcomings, we can be our own harshest critics. However, mindfulness teaches us to observe our experiences without the need for judgment or self-criticism.

Self-compassion during the reflective process allows us to acknowledge our imperfections without condemning ourselves. It's a reminder that we are human and that growth is a process. Mistakes and setbacks are opportunities for learning, not reasons for punishment. By treating ourselves with compassion, we remove the barriers that prevent us from fully understanding and embracing our experiences. This compassionate approach encourages emotional healing and fosters a more positive, supportive relationship with ourselves.

Self-Reflection From a Place of Curiosity

Curiosity plays a vital role in both self-reflection and mindfulness. Mindfulness encourages us to be curious about our present experience—about the sensations, thoughts, and feelings that arise in the moment. Curiosity can enhance our process of self-reflection, allowing us to explore our inner world with an open mind.

When we reflect mindfully, we are less likely to jump to conclusions or rush to fix our problems. Instead, we remain open and curious, asking ourselves questions such as, "What is this experience teaching me?" or "What does this feeling tell me about myself?" By approaching our reflections with curiosity, we open ourselves to new insights and a deeper understanding of our emotional landscape.

Curiosity allows us to move beyond surface-level reflections, helping us explore the root causes of our thoughts and behaviors. Instead of simply acknowledging that we feel anxious or frustrated, we dig deeper to understand why. What are the underlying fears or beliefs that fuel these emotions? How can we address them in a way that promotes growth? Curiosity enables us to discover these layers of understanding, leading to more profound self-awareness.

Integrating Mindfulness and Reflection

By combining mindfulness and self-reflection, we gain deeper insights into who we are and why we do what we do. This awareness is essential for making intentional changes in our lives.

Through mindful self-reflection, we can identify areas where we may want to grow. Whether we seek to improve our relationships, become more resilient, or develop a deeper sense of purpose, mindfulness helps us approach these changes with clarity and intention. We are better able to assess our strengths and areas for improvement, and with self-compassion, we can create a path forward that aligns with our values and goals.

Mindfulness also helps us stay grounded in the present moment as we work toward our personal growth. It encourages us to focus on the process rather than rushing toward an outcome. Personal growth is not a destination but a continuous journey. By integrating mindfulness into self-reflection, we can stay connected to that journey, embracing each step along the way.

Moving Forward with Insight and Intention

Mindful self-reflection doesn't just help us understand ourselves in the present; it also informs how we move forward. With greater self-awareness, we can make decisions that are more aligned with our values and desires. We approach life with greater clarity, intentionality, and a deeper sense of purpose.

Reflecting mindfully allows us to see patterns in our behavior and make conscious decisions to change them. It provides us with the insight to understand what drives us, what serves us, and what we might need to leave behind. By practicing mindfulness in our reflections, we can continue to evolve, making thoughtful choices that lead to a more fulfilling and authentic life.

Receiving Greater Clarity and Understanding

Mindfulness and self-reflection are powerful tools for personal growth and emotional well-being. Mindfulness cultivates awareness and clarity, while self-reflection provides the opportunity to understand ourselves more deeply. Together, these practices create a space where we can examine our thoughts, emotions, and behaviors with compassion and curiosity, fostering deeper insights and greater self-awareness. Through mindful self-reflection, we can move forward with intention, embrace personal growth, and navigate life with greater clarity and understanding.

CHAPTER 28: MINDFUL JOURNALING

Journaling is an effective tool that encourages awareness and introspection. When practiced mindfully, it becomes more than just a way to record events or thoughts. It becomes a method to engage with the present moment, to observe our internal landscape with care and focus, and to gain insight into our emotional and mental patterns. Mindful journaling is not about producing a polished result or conforming to a set of expectations—it is about the experience of writing itself.

This chapter will explore how the practice of mindful journaling supports mental clarity and emotional insight, offering a structured approach to writing that nurtures self-awareness and reflection. It focuses on the process of writing, where each moment of reflection and each word written contributes to a deeper understanding of the self.

Setting the Scene

Before you begin journaling, it is important to create a space that allows for focus and reflection. This can be done in any environment where you feel comfortable enough to sit quietly with your thoughts. While the setting itself doesn't need to be extravagant or formal, the goal is to remove distractions and create a space where your attention can remain with the process of writing.

You might choose a quiet corner of your home, a park bench,

or even a spot by a window that allows you to focus. The key is to be in a space that encourages your mind to settle and your thoughts to surface freely. This isn't about creating the "perfect" writing environment—rather, it is about cultivating a setting that allows you to engage fully with the present moment.

Once you've found your space, take a few moments to center yourself. Simply being present in the moment, without rushing to begin, can shift your mindset and prepare you for mindful reflection.

Engaging with the Present

Mindful journaling is a way of slowing down and paying attention to what is unfolding in your mind. The purpose of this practice is to engage with the present moment and allow your thoughts to flow naturally, without judgment or expectation.

When you write mindfully, you do not have to worry about whether your sentences are complete or whether your ideas are well-formed. You can simply allow whatever is present in your mind to take shape on the page. This means there is no pressure to edit or revise in the moment. Instead, you can observe your thoughts and let them flow freely and spill out as they come.

As you write, you may notice patterns in your thinking. You may find certain themes, emotions, or experiences reappearing. This is a natural part of the process. Mindful journaling offers a chance to recognize these patterns without needing to "fix" them. You can simply allow them to exist and observe them with curiosity. Over time, this practice encourages a deeper awareness of your mental and emotional processes, providing clarity and insight into what occupies your mind.

The Process of Observation Through Writing

At the heart of mindful journaling is the act of observation. You do not have to write to follow a certain format or achieve a specific outcome. Instead, you can write to become more aware of what is happening with your thoughts and feelings. Writing in this way helps you observe your inner experience from a fresh perspective. Journaling encourages you to step back and view your emotions, ideas, and experiences as they are instead of engaging in automatic thinking or reacting to situations

In this process, there is no need to alter your thoughts or feelings. You are simply acknowledging them as they arise and recording them. By bringing your attention to the present moment through writing, you allow the complexity of your internal world to be expressed in its natural form. There is no need to "clean it up" or modify it to fit any expectation. By accepting your thoughts in their raw state, you build a clearer understanding of how your own mind works.

Gaining Insight into Thought Patterns

One of the most valuable aspects of mindful journaling is the ability to track and observe your recurring thought patterns. Over time, as you write regularly, you may begin to notice certain thoughts that keep arising. These might include worries, concerns, hopes, or unresolved emotions. Identifying these patterns can lead to greater clarity about the aspects of life that influence your thoughts and feelings.

Mindful journaling allows you to become aware of your mental habits—those repetitive thought cycles that can take up a significant portion of your mental energy. By noticing these patterns, you can begin to understand the underlying beliefs or assumptions that may be shaping your perspective. This level of awareness is the first step toward making conscious changes, should you choose to do so.

The practice of observing these patterns in your journal allows you to document your emotional states and identify triggers that cause particular responses. This awareness provides an opportunity to respond to challenges with a clearer understanding of the underlying causes of your emotions. Over time, journaling offers a way to track emotional growth and discover areas that require more attention or reflection.

Writing as a Tool for Problem Solving

Journaling can also serve as a practical tool for solving problems or gaining increased clarity in difficult situations. When faced with a challenge, writing can help organize thoughts and ideas that may feel fragmented in the mind. The act of writing allows you to approach the issue from a more structured perspective, bringing a sense of order to otherwise overwhelming circumstances.

By writing about a problem, you create the space to articulate its various aspects, helping you explore different solutions or perspectives. As you journal about the situation, your thoughts may become clearer, and you may gain new insights that weren't immediately apparent when you first encountered the issue. The process of writing helps break down complex situations into manageable pieces, enabling you to look at them from different angles.

This doesn't mean that you will necessarily find immediate answers or solutions. Rather, mindful journaling offers a way to sit with the uncertainty and explore the situation more deeply, helping you make decisions that align with your values or desired outcomes.

Reflecting on Emotions Without Attachment

Writing mindfully encourages you to engage with your emotions in a way that fosters understanding and detachment. Emotions often arise and pass through us in waves, sometimes leaving us feeling overwhelmed or unsettled. Mindful journaling offers a space to reflect on these emotions without becoming attached to them.

You might write about how you're feeling in the moment, expressing frustration, joy, sadness, or confusion. These emotions do not need to be fixed or analyzed immediately. Instead, the act of journaling gives you the opportunity to acknowledge these feelings, recognize them for what they are, and allow them to exist without judgment. This practice encourages emotional clarity and helps prevent you from getting lost in your emotions or reacting impulsively to them.

In this way, mindful journaling acts as an emotional outlet, a way to express and examine your feelings without becoming overwhelmed. It allows you to sit with your emotions, not as a way to change them, but as a means of simply observing them.

Building a Habit of Self-Reflection

Mindful journaling is most effective when practiced regularly. By writing consistently, you create a habit of self-reflection that encourages ongoing awareness and insight. This doesn't mean journaling every day, but rather making it a part of your routine in a way that feels right for you.

As you develop this habit, you may notice subtle changes in your thinking. Over time, regular journaling allows you to track the evolution of your thoughts, emotions, and responses. You may begin to notice shifts in perspective, or discover new ways of dealing with challenges or stressors.

The consistency of journaling supports the development of a reflective mindset. Each time you write, you are cultivating an ongoing process of self-awareness. This habitual practice deepens your connection with your inner thoughts and creates space for growth, helping you observe and respond to life's challenges with greater clarity and presence.

Writing for Clarity and Understanding

Ultimately, the purpose of mindful journaling is to provide clarity. In a world where thoughts can sometimes feel jumbled and disconnected, journaling offers a way to bring structure and order to your internal dialogue. It offers a method for organizing your thoughts, clarifying emotions, and gaining insight into your life.

As you journal, you might notice that things become clearer over time. Writing about a situation or an emotion allows you to articulate it in a way that makes sense. What once felt confusing or overwhelming may, through the process of writing, become more understandable and manageable.

In this sense, journaling provides not only a means of reflection but also a tool for decision-making, emotional processing, and problem-solving. The act of putting thoughts into words is often enough to bring clarity, and the ongoing practice of writing encourages a steady focus on the present moment.

A Space for Reflection and Clarity

Mindful journaling is a simple yet profound practice that provides a space for reflection, emotional awareness, and mental clarity. By engaging with the act of writing with full attention and presence, you allow your thoughts and feelings to unfold naturally, without pressure or expectation. In doing so, you gain insight into your inner world, track patterns in your thinking and emotions, and clarify your responses to various situations.

This practice, when approached regularly and without judgment, helps foster greater self-awareness and personal growth. Writing mindfully is an effective way to build a clearer understanding of your experiences and to reflect on the complexities of your emotions, offering an ongoing dialogue with yourself that brings peace, understanding, and insight.

CHAPTER 29: UNLOCKING YOUR POWER THROUGH MINDFULNESS

Mindfulness can hold the key to unlocking your personal power. By being fully aware of the present moment—without judgment or distraction—it allows us to tap into our inherent strength, clarity, and authenticity. In this state of awareness, we connect with our true self, not as a product of our past experiences or future expectations, but as an individual with the capacity to create, choose, and act with intention.

The act of being mindful creates a space where we can recognize our own agency. It helps us step away from habitual reactions, mental distractions, and emotional turbulence, offering the chance to embrace life with a greater sense of empowerment and control. By fostering this awareness, mindfulness enables us to unlock a power that is not driven by external forces but is inherent in our ability to observe, reflect, and choose how to engage with the world.

Mindfulness: A Gateway to Self-Mastery

At its core, mindfulness is the art of living with intention and presence. It is the ability to engage with each moment fully, without judgment, expectation, or distraction. When we practice mindfulness, we are not trying to change who we are; instead, we become more attuned to our thoughts, feelings, and sensations. This heightened awareness creates the foundation for self-mastery—the ability to respond to life with calm, clarity, and purpose.

Self-mastery is not about controlling every aspect of our lives. Rather, it is about understanding ourselves deeply enough to recognize when we are being influenced by unconscious patterns, automatic reactions, or external pressures. Through mindfulness, we begin to notice when we are acting out of habit, fear, or insecurity, and we gain the power to shift our response. Mindfulness empowers us to break free from ways of thinking and behaving that no longer serve us and choose how we want to act, based on what we truly want and value.

The Power of Self-Awareness

One of the most profound ways mindfulness unlocks our power is through self-awareness. Self-awareness allows us to see ourselves clearly, without the distortion of judgment, expectation, or self-criticism. Most of the time, we are not fully aware of our thoughts and feelings. They arise automatically, without our conscious input, and we react to them without questioning whether they are true, helpful, or aligned with our deepest values.

Mindfulness offers us the opportunity to pause and observe our internal landscape. It creates a space between stimulus and response, allowing us to witness our thoughts and feelings as they arise. In this space, we can choose how to respond rather than being swept away by our automatic reactions. Self-awareness is the first step toward empowerment because it gives us the ability to see ourselves clearly and make decisions from a place of understanding, rather than blind reaction or emotional impulse.

Through mindfulness, we become more aware of our beliefs about ourselves and others, the assumptions we hold, and the habitual ways we respond to situations. We begin to understand our motivations and triggers, and this understanding gives us the ability to make conscious choices. Instead of being controlled by unconscious biases or ingrained habits, we can become active participants in our own lives, choosing the actions and responses that align with who we truly want to be.

Embracing the Present Moment

True Power resides in the present moment. Too often, we allow ourselves to be consumed by past regrets or future anxieties. We worry about things that may never happen, replay past mistakes, or envision negative outcomes. While these thoughts are natural, they often prevent us from fully engaging with the present, where our power to create, decide, and act exists.

Mindfulness is a practice of bringing our full attention to the present moment. When we focus on the now, we stop getting lost in mental chatter or emotional turbulence. Instead of being carried away by memories or projections, we tune into the reality of the current moment. In doing so, we experience life as it is, with greater clarity, perspective, and purpose. This heightened awareness connects us to the moment, and in turn, to our own capacity to make clear and intentional decisions.

When we are fully present, we are no longer distracted by worries about the future or the past. We see things as they are, and we are able to respond with a calm and balanced mind. This ability to be present is empowering because it allows us to engage with life from a place of centeredness. We are no longer at the mercy of external circumstances, emotional reactions, or automatic patterns. We can choose how to act, based on what truly matters to us in the here and now.

The Role of Acceptance in Unlocking Power

One of the key tenets of mindfulness is acceptance. Acceptance does not mean resigning ourselves to situations or giving up on personal growth. Rather, it is about acknowledging things as they are—without judgment or resistance. Acceptance allows us to stop fighting against reality, which only creates unnecessary stress and frustration. It is the recognition that while we may not always be able to control external circumstances, we can always control how we choose to respond.

Mindfulness helps us to release these unrealistic expectations. It teaches us that we are enough as we are, without needing to prove ourselves or meet external standards. By accepting ourselves in our entirety—including our flaws and weaknesses—we unlock a deep sense of peace and power that comes from being authentic and true to who we are.

When we accept ourselves, we also accept life's challenges, knowing that they are a natural part of growth and change. Instead of resisting difficulty, we embrace it as an opportunity to learn, grow, and become more resilient. This acceptance is liberating, as it frees us from the weight of disempowerment and self-criticism. It allows us to move through life with greater ease, confidence, and clarity, knowing that we have the ability to navigate whatever comes our way.

Letting Go of Limiting Beliefs

Another aspect of unlocking our power through mindfulness is the process of letting go of limiting beliefs. Many of us carry deeply ingrained ideas about who we are and what we are capable of. These beliefs often arise from past experiences, social conditioning, or cultural norms, and they can limit our potential in ways we are not always aware of.

Mindfulness helps us become aware of these limiting beliefs by allowing us to observe our thoughts without judgment. As we practice mindfulness, we begin to recognize the stories we tell ourselves about our abilities, our worth, and our limitations. We start to question whether these beliefs are true or helpful, and we gain the power to let go of those that no longer serve us.

Letting go of limiting beliefs opens up space for growth, creativity, and possibility. It allows us to break free from the constraints we've placed on ourselves and move beyond the boundaries of our own self-imposed limitations. By letting go of these beliefs, we empower ourselves to take risks, try new things, and step into the unknown with confidence and courage. Through mindfulness, we unlock the full range of our potential and begin to live in alignment with our true capabilities.

Building Confidence Through Mindfulness

Mindfulness is also a powerful tool for building confidence. Confidence is not something that can be manufactured or forced; it is a natural byproduct of self-awareness, acceptance, and trust. When we practice mindfulness, we develop a deeper connection to ourselves, which in turn strengthens our confidence. We begin to trust ourselves more because we understand our thoughts, emotions, and needs on a deeper level. We recognize our strengths, acknowledge our weaknesses, and embrace both as parts of our authentic self.

This confidence is not based on external validation, but on an inner sense of self-assurance that comes from being present, aware, and true to who we are. As we build this self-trust, we begin to approach life's challenges with greater courage and resilience. Instead of fearing failure or judgment, we embrace the process of growth and self-discovery. We know that whatever happens, we have the ability to learn, adapt, and move forward with clarity and strength.

The Power of Choice

One of the greatest sources of power that mindfulness provides is the ability to choose how we respond to life. In any given moment, we have the power to decide how to react to our thoughts, emotions, and experiences. We are not victims of circumstance or slaves to our emotions. Through mindfulness, we become more attuned to our internal state and more aware of the choices available to us.

Instead of automatically reacting to situations or acting out of habit, mindfulness allows us to pause, reflect, and choose our response. This ability to make conscious choices empowers us to take control of our lives and shape our experiences. Whether it's making decisions about our relationships, our career, or our personal growth, mindfulness gives us the clarity and confidence to choose actions that align with our goals and values.

A Dynamic and Transformative Practice

Mindfulness is not a passive practice; it is a dynamic and transformative tool that unlocks our inherent power. By cultivating self-awareness, acceptance, and presence, we can step into a place of clarity and confidence. Mindfulness teaches us to observe our thoughts, feelings, and behaviors without judgment, allowing us to make conscious choices that reflect our true values. Through mindfulness, we release limiting beliefs, embrace our imperfections, and build a deep sense of trust in ourselves.

As we unlock our power through mindfulness, we gain the ability to live intentionally, with purpose and authenticity. We become the authors of our own lives, no longer bound by the unconscious patterns that have shaped us in the past. Mindfulness allows us to step into our full potential, making empowered choices that align with our deepest aspirations and values. In this way, mindfulness becomes not just a practice, but a way of life—one that is centered, empowered, and truly our own.

CHAPTER 30: MINDFULNESS FOR PERSONAL GROWTH AND TRANSFORMATION

Mindfulness, often thought of as a method for increasing moment-to-moment awareness, also holds immense potential to assist with personal growth and transformation. At its core, mindfulness offers a way to observe and engage with our experiences without judgment, allowing us to develop a deeper understanding of ourselves. This awareness becomes the foundation for change, enabling us to break free from limiting patterns, challenge old habits, and create new behaviors that better align with our authentic values and aspirations.

Personal growth is not a linear journey, and transformation does not happen overnight. It is, however, a process—a journey of gradual unfolding where we learn more about who we are, what we truly desire, and how we can cultivate a life that reflects our deepest truths. Mindfulness serves as a gentle yet powerful companion along this path, helping us build awareness, cultivate intentionality, and make thoughtful choices that lead to meaningful change.

The Role of Mindfulness in Self-Awareness

Self-awareness is the cornerstone of personal growth. Without truly understanding ourselves—the patterns that shape our behavior, the beliefs that inform our decisions, and the emotions that guide our reactions—change is difficult to achieve. Mindfulness offers a way to access this deeper self-awareness by bringing our attention to the present moment. Rather than reacting automatically to situations, mindfulness invites us to observe our thoughts, emotions, and actions with clarity and without judgment.

Through mindfulness, we become more attuned to our habitual ways of thinking and behaving. We may start to notice patterns in how we respond to stress, how we interact with others, or how we handle difficult emotions. Often, these patterns are so ingrained in our lives that we are not fully conscious of them. Mindfulness allows us to observe them from a place of detachment, creating the space to reflect on whether these patterns are serving us or hindering our growth.

For instance, we may discover that we have a tendency to procrastinate when faced with certain tasks or that we react defensively in challenging conversations. Instead of simply accepting these behaviors as part of who we are, mindfulness gives us the awareness to recognize them and choose a different response. With this awareness comes the power to change—slowly, over time—as we practice new ways of being in the world.

Breaking Old Patterns and Creating New Habits

One of the most profound benefits of mindfulness is its ability to help us break free from old patterns of thinking, feeling, and behaving. Over time, we all develop habits, some of which serve us well, while others may limit our potential. Whether it's a negative self-talk pattern, a fixed mindset, or a way of handling conflict that causes more harm than good, mindfulness gives us the clarity to see these habits for what they are.

When we approach personal growth with mindfulness, we

begin to recognize the stories we tell ourselves—the limiting beliefs that keep us stuck in old patterns. These beliefs may have formed early in our lives, often as a way of protecting ourselves or making sense of the world. Yet, as we grow and evolve, these old beliefs can prevent us from reaching our full potential.

Through mindful awareness, we can start to challenge these beliefs. Instead of automatically accepting the story that we are "not good enough" or "incapable of change," mindfulness encourages us to question those thoughts. By simply noticing them without attaching to them, we open up the possibility of transformation. With consistent mindfulness practice, we begin to create new beliefs and habits that are aligned with our true values and aspirations.

For example, if we notice a recurring thought of inadequacy in our work, mindfulness can help us step back and view this thought objectively. Rather than believing it as truth, we can ask ourselves: Is this thought helpful? Is it reflective of who I truly am? Over time, mindfulness empowers us to create new, more empowering thoughts that replace old, unhelpful ones. This gradual process of change allows us to break free from limiting patterns and embrace a more positive and empowered way of living.

Cultivating New, Empowering Habits

Personal growth is often associated with developing new habits —habits that align with our values and support our long-term goals. Mindfulness can play a crucial role in this process by helping us become more intentional about the habits we want to cultivate. It provides the awareness to observe our current habits and assess whether they are aligned with who we want to become.

Habits, whether positive or negative, are often formed through repetition. By paying attention to our thoughts, actions, and motivations in a mindful way, we can start to notice the patterns that govern our behavior. Mindfulness offers a moment-to-moment awareness that helps us interrupt automatic reactions and make more conscious choices. Over time, this conscious decision-making process allows us to create habits that are more supportive of our personal growth.

For instance, if we want to cultivate the habit of exercising regularly, mindfulness can help us notice when we are making excuses or when our mind starts to create barriers to taking action. With mindfulness, we can observe these thoughts and choose a different course of action. By simply noticing the resistance and moving through it, we begin to establish new habits that align with our goals.

This process of cultivating new habits through mindfulness doesn't have to be overwhelming. Instead of trying to overhaul every aspect of our lives all at once, mindfulness encourages us to focus on one area at a time. Whether it's dedicating time to a creative pursuit, setting aside space for reflection, or practicing patience in our interactions, mindfulness allows us to build habits that are grounded in intention and self-awareness.

Rewriting of Stories

One of the most powerful ways mindfulness supports personal growth is by helping us rewrite the stories we have been telling ourselves. These stories, often based on past experiences, can shape how we see ourselves and the world around us. Sometimes, these narratives are limiting, keeping us stuck in patterns of fear, self-doubt, or unfulfilled potential.

Mindfulness offers the space to pause and become aware of these stories. Instead of mindlessly replaying old narratives, we begin to notice the impact these stories have on our behavior and choices. In this space of awareness, we can choose to rewrite the story.

For example, we may have an old story about failure that holds us back from pursuing new opportunities. By practicing mindfulness, we observe this story without getting swept away by it. We notice its grip and decide that we no longer want to carry that story forward. This practice allows us to write a new story—one that acknowledges our strengths, our growth, and our ability to handle challenges with resilience.

Mindfulness enables us to break free from old patterns and create a more empowering narrative for ourselves. It encourages us to see ourselves as active participants in the process of change, capable of rewriting the stories that no longer serve us. In this way, mindfulness acts as a transformative tool, allowing us to break free from the past and step into the present with a sense of possibility and empowerment.

Mindfulness and Emotional Intelligence

Another area where mindfulness significantly contributes to personal growth is in the cultivation of emotional intelligence. Emotional intelligence is the ability to understand, manage, and express emotions effectively. Mindfulness enhances our emotional intelligence by helping us become more aware of our emotional states and how they influence our behavior.

Through mindfulness, we develop the ability to observe our emotions as they arise, without being overwhelmed by them. This awareness allows us to respond to emotions in a thoughtful and constructive way, rather than reacting impulsively. As we become more mindful of our emotions, we learn to recognize patterns in how we experience and express them. We become better at navigating difficult emotions, such as anger, frustration, or sadness, and are able to handle them in a way that is aligned with our values and goals.

Mindfulness also helps us develop greater empathy and compassion for others. By cultivating awareness of our own emotional states, we become more attuned to the emotions of those around us. This increased emotional intelligence allows us to connect with others more deeply, foster healthier relationships, and navigate social interactions with greater sensitivity.

The Continuous Nature of Personal Growth

Personal growth is not a destination—it is an ongoing process. Just as mindfulness is a practice that requires consistent attention and awareness, personal growth is a continuous journey of self-discovery and transformation. There are always new layers of awareness to uncover, new patterns to break, and new habits to cultivate.

Mindfulness helps us embrace this process with patience and compassion, allowing us to grow at our own pace. Instead of seeking immediate results or trying to force change, mindfulness teaches us to stay present with where we are and trust that growth will unfold naturally. We do not need to be perfect, and we do not need to have all the answers. Mindfulness reminds us that the journey itself is just as valuable as the destination.

Through mindfulness, we begin to see that personal growth is not about becoming someone we are not but about uncovering who we truly are. It is about peeling back the layers of conditioning and self-doubt to reveal the authentic self underneath. With each mindful step, we grow in self-awareness, self-acceptance, and self-empowerment.

Mindfulness and Transformation

Mindfulness is vital to personal growth and transformation. By fostering self-awareness, breaking old patterns, and cultivating new empowering habits, mindfulness allows us to step into a life that aligns with our values and aspirations. It helps us rewrite the stories we've been telling ourselves and develop the emotional intelligence necessary to navigate our relationships and interactions with others.

Personal growth is not an overnight achievement, but a continuous process—a journey that requires patience, presence, and practice. Mindfulness offers us the space and clarity to move through this journey with intention, self-compassion, and openness to change. As we engage in mindfulness practice, we unlock the potential for profound transformation, guiding us toward a life that is authentic, meaningful, and fully aligned with who we are meant to be.

CHAPTER 31: LIVING WITH PURPOSE AND PRESENCE

The path to discovering and sustaining purpose is often complex and, at times, elusive. Purpose gives our lives direction, meaning, and a sense of fulfillment. It allows us to act with intention, to make decisions that reflect our values, and to move forward with confidence in our unique direction. However, while purpose can guide us toward a meaningful existence, it is not always something that can be fixed in time—it is a fluid concept, changing and evolving as we move through different phases of life.

Mindfulness is a tool that can help us navigate this journey toward purposeful living. By anchoring ourselves in the present moment, we not only make more intentional choices but also discover what truly matters to us. Living with purpose is not only about grand goals and aspirations, but also about the alignment of our day-to-day actions with our deeper values. When we live with intention and mindfulness, we open ourselves to the full richness of the moment, cultivating a life that is meaningful, fulfilling, and authentic.

Purposeful Living: The Heart of Mindfulness

Purposeful living starts with clarity—a deep understanding of who we are, what we stand for, and what we truly want to experience in our lives. Purpose is not simply about setting goals; it's about understanding the driving force behind those goals and allowing our actions to reflect our core values. Too often, we go through life reacting to circumstances rather than consciously choosing how we want to engage with the world around us. In the absence of mindfulness, we might follow external expectations or drift into autopilot, forgetting to check in with ourselves to see if our actions align with our inner desires.

Mindfulness brings us into the present moment with intention, allowing us to observe our thoughts, feelings, and behaviors. With this awareness, we can begin to ask ourselves: "Is this action in alignment with my values?" "Does this decision bring me closer to the life I want to create?" These questions form the foundation of mindful, purposeful living. Rather than acting on impulse or habit, mindfulness invites us to slow down and check in with our deeper selves.

Through mindful reflection, we can examine our core values—whether it's integrity, creativity, kindness, or any other value—and assess how well we are living in accordance with them. Mindfulness helps us peel back the layers of distraction and noise in our lives, giving us the clarity to make choices that reflect our true selves. In doing so, we align our actions with our purpose, leading to a more fulfilling and authentic existence.

Mindfulness as a Tool for Clarity

Clarity is a crucial element of purposeful living. Without it, we may feel lost, uncertain, or overwhelmed by the many demands and expectations placed on us. Mindfulness helps us cut through the noise of daily life by encouraging us to stay present, focused, and attuned to our inner world. When we practice mindfulness, we engage fully with our current experience, which allows us to step back from the rush of external influences and gain a clearer perspective on what truly matters.

In the quiet space that mindfulness creates, we can more easily distinguish between what is truly important to us and what might be a fleeting distraction. When our minds are cluttered with unimportant details or we are preoccupied with the opinions of others, we lose touch with our purpose. Mindfulness creates the mental space needed to sift through this clutter and bring attention to what is meaningful.

For example, in a moment of mindfulness, we might notice that we've been prioritizing things that don't really serve us, like constantly striving to meet the expectations of others or giving undue attention to things that are ultimately trivial. By being mindful of these patterns, we gain the clarity to make adjustments, to shift our focus back to what truly matters. This ability to tune in to our own inner compass allows us to navigate life with a greater sense of direction and intention.

Clarity doesn't necessarily mean having all the answers, but it does allow us to recognize the next right step. It's the ability to know, deep down, when we are moving closer to or further away from our true aspirations. Through mindfulness, we develop the ability to discern what aligns with our authentic desires and make decisions from a place of deep awareness rather than reaction or external influence.

Living in the Moment with Purpose

While clarity is essential for purposeful living, so is presence. Mindfulness teaches us that while long-term goals and aspirations are important, it is in the present moment where true fulfillment resides. So often, we become consumed with thoughts of the future or regrets about the past, forgetting that the only moment we truly have is the one we are experiencing right now.

Living in the present moment with purpose does not mean that we abandon our long-term goals or neglect the future—it simply means that we engage fully with the current moment, understanding that the actions we take today shape our tomorrow. Each step we take, no matter how small, contributes to the larger picture of our lives. When we are fully present, we are able to bring intention to each moment, which makes every experience richer and more meaningful.

Consider how often we rush through daily tasks, from eating to working to interacting with others, without really engaging with the experience itself. Mindfulness encourages us to slow down and immerse ourselves fully in what we are doing. Whether it's savoring the taste of food, giving our full attention to a conversation, or focusing completely on a creative endeavor, mindfulness brings us into the moment and allows us to live with purpose in every action.

In this way, mindfulness doesn't simply help us move through life's tasks but also enriches our experience of them. Even mundane activities become opportunities for purposeful living when we are present with them. When we are mindful of how we engage with each task, we bring more meaning to what we do, and in turn, to the life we create.

Intentional Choices: Aligning Action with Values

At the heart of mindfulness is the ability to make intentional choices. Instead of reacting impulsively or habitually, mindfulness gives us the clarity to choose how we respond to life's challenges and opportunities. Every choice, big or small, is an opportunity to align our actions with our values and goals.

The process of making intentional choices begins with awareness. By noticing our thoughts, emotions, and tendencies, we can recognize when we are being pulled in directions that do not reflect our deepest desires. Mindfulness helps us step back, observe the situation, and ask: "Is this choice in alignment with my purpose?" "Will this action bring me closer to the life I want to live?"

When we approach life with mindfulness, we recognize that every decision is a chance to create the life we want. We stop reacting from a place of fear, habit, or external pressure, and instead, we choose actions that reflect our true intentions. Mindfulness also allows us to check in with ourselves regularly, so we can course-correct when necessary.

For example, if we find ourselves consistently overcommitting to tasks that do not align with our purpose, mindfulness provides us with the opportunity to step back and reassess. By noticing this pattern, we can make more intentional choices that are in line with our values, whether it's saying no to an obligation or setting aside time for a more fulfilling activity.

Through mindfulness, we build a habit of reflecting on our choices and ensuring that our actions are purposeful and aligned with our long-term vision. This creates a ripple effect, where each intentional choice we make reinforces our sense of purpose and direction.

Living with Both Purpose and Presence

Purpose and presence are not opposing forces; they are deeply interconnected. Purpose provides us with direction and meaning, while presence allows us to experience the richness of each moment. By living with both purpose and presence, we create a life that is both intentional and fulfilling.

Mindfulness teaches us that purpose is not just a future goal to be attained, but something that can be woven into the fabric of our daily lives. We do not need to wait for the future to be purposeful—we can choose to live with purpose in every moment. Similarly, presence does not mean neglecting our long-term goals; it simply means that we recognize the importance of the journey itself and take each step mindfully, with intention.

When we live with both purpose and presence, we deepen our connection to ourselves and to the world around us. We engage more fully with each experience, make choices that are aligned with our true desires, and create a life that reflects our deepest values. We discover that the present moment, fully lived, is the most powerful vehicle for creating the future we desire.

A Continuous Practice

Living with purpose and presence is not a destination but a continuous practice. It is about making intentional choices, aligning our actions with our values, and remaining fully engaged in each moment. Through mindfulness, we gain clarity about what truly matters to us and create a life that reflects our deepest desires. When we live with both purpose and presence, we experience a profound sense of fulfillment and connection, knowing that each moment is a chance to live in alignment with our highest aspirations.

As we navigate this journey, mindfulness empowers us to stay grounded in the present while moving toward a future that is meaningful and intentional. It is through the integration of purpose and presence that we create lives of greater authenticity, satisfaction, and joy.

CHAPTER 32: MOVING FORWARD WITH MINDFULNESS

Mindfulness is a practice that empowers us to engage with life more fully, to embrace each moment with clarity, awareness, and purpose. It is a way of being that enables us to meet the complexities of life with greater ease and insight. Mindfulness a continuous and evolving practice, offering the possibility of deeper understanding and profound transformation over time.

As we look to the future, we realize that mindfulness is not something to be sought for a fleeting moment or applied only in times of difficulty. It is a pathway that can enrich every aspect of our lives, providing us with the tools to navigate change, respond to challenges, and live with intention and presence. As we continue our journey, mindfulness becomes a powerful companion—one that helps us stay grounded, centered, and resilient no matter what arises.

Mindfulness in a Changing World

The world is in a constant state of flux. Our lives, our relationships, and our circumstances shift in ways we can't always anticipate. In many cases, change can seem overwhelming, unpredictable, and beyond our control. Yet, mindfulness offers us a way to stay anchored amidst this fluidity. It gives us the ability to experience the present moment without clinging to the past or grasping for a future that is yet to come.

By cultivating mindfulness, we learn to observe change without being swept away by it. We begin to see that change does not always have to be feared or resisted; rather, it can be embraced as part of the natural ebb and flow of life. Mindfulness teaches us how to approach change with curiosity and openness, welcoming the unknown with a sense of readiness and calm. It reminds us that, although external circumstances may be unpredictable, we always have the power to choose how we respond.

As we move through life, we often encounter moments of uncertainty—times when the path forward is unclear, or when we feel uncertain about the choices we are making. Mindfulness helps us meet these moments with clarity, allowing us to pause and reflect before taking action. It enables us to notice our thoughts and emotions as they arise, giving us space to decide how to respond rather than reacting impulsively or out of habit. In doing so, mindfulness fosters a sense of agency and control over how we navigate life's twists and turns.

Mindfulness also allows us to develop resilience in the face of change. Rather than viewing challenges as obstacles, mindfulness invites us to approach them as opportunities for growth. When we cultivate mindfulness, we learn to adapt to shifting circumstances with grace and ease, knowing that change, while sometimes difficult, is an inevitable part of life's journey. By staying grounded and present, we are able to weather life's storms without being overwhelmed, and to emerge from them with a greater sense of understanding and strength.

The Hope for a Mindful Future

Looking ahead, mindfulness offers a hopeful vision for the future. This vision is not about perfection or a life free of challenges, but rather about creating a future where mindfulness serves as a guiding principle—one that brings clarity, peace, and presence to every moment. This future is built on a foundation of mindful awareness, where individuals are empowered to live with intention, connect deeply with themselves, and engage with the world around them in ways that are authentic and meaningful.

The beauty of mindfulness lies in its ability to transcend the personal and ripple outward. When we embrace mindfulness in our own lives, it naturally affects the way we interact with others. By cultivating a more mindful approach to our own experiences, we become better able to listen, understand, and connect with those around us. We bring more compassion, patience, and empathy to our relationships, creating deeper bonds and more harmonious interactions.

In a world that can often feel fragmented and disconnected, mindfulness provides a way to bridge the gap. It encourages us to step away from distractions and engage more fully with the people and experiences around us. When we are truly present, we are able to listen attentively, speak with intention, and engage in relationships with a sense of clarity and respect. This presence creates the foundation for deeper connection and a greater sense of belonging, not just for ourselves, but for others as well.

Mindfulness also allows us to live more in alignment with our own values and aspirations. It helps us to clear away the noise of external pressures and to tune into what truly matters. When we are mindful, we are more likely to make choices that reflect our deepest desires and intentions, rather than acting out of habit or societal expectation. As a result, we begin to create lives that are not just successful by external standards, but deeply fulfilling on a personal level.

In envisioning a mindful future, we see a world where individuals, guided by their own awareness, make choices that foster personal well-being, social harmony, and a deep sense of purpose. This mindful future is one where each moment is lived with intention, each decision is made with clarity, and each interaction is grounded in presence and understanding.

The Journey of Mindfulness

Mindfulness is not a destination, but a continuous journey. It is a practice that deepens over time, unfolding in layers as we become more attuned to our thoughts, emotions, and experiences. Each day, each moment, offers us the opportunity to engage more fully with the present. And in doing so, we find that the journey itself is the destination.

The practice of mindfulness begins with small, simple steps. At first, it may seem like just a momentary pause, a brief respite from the demands of life. But as we continue to practice, we begin to see that mindfulness is not something we can compartmentalize or isolate—it is a way of being that permeates every aspect of our lives. Whether we are washing dishes, taking a walk, or having a conversation, mindfulness invites us to be fully present, to bring our full attention and awareness to whatever we are doing.

Over time, mindfulness allows us to gain deeper insight into our own patterns and tendencies. We begin to notice how we react to situations, how we respond to stress, and how we engage with our emotions. This awareness is the first step in transformation. By simply noticing our thoughts and behaviors without judgment, we create the space for change. We start to see how our habits and reactions may no longer serve us, and we begin to make different choices. Through this process of awareness, we cultivate the capacity to break free from old patterns and create new, more empowering ways of thinking and being.

Mindfulness also brings us closer to our values and aspirations. By slowing down and being present, we are able to discern what is truly important to us. In our busy lives, it is easy to become distracted by external pressures or superficial goals. Mindfulness helps us to reconnect with our deeper desires, guiding us toward lives that are more in alignment with our authentic selves. It encourages us to make choices that reflect our values, allowing us to create lives that are meaningful and fulfilling.

The journey of mindfulness is one of discovery. With each step, we uncover more about ourselves and the world around us. We become more attuned to the richness of life, noticing the small details that we might otherwise overlook. Mindfulness helps us to see the beauty in the mundane, to appreciate the present moment for what it is, and to engage with life with a sense of wonder and curiosity.

As we continue on this journey, we find that mindfulness becomes less of a practice and more of a way of life. It informs our decisions, our relationships, and our sense of self. It helps us to stay grounded, present, and aware as we move through the various stages and experiences of life. And with each moment of mindfulness, we become more attuned to the fullness of our own lives, living with greater intention, clarity, and purpose.

Mindfulness as an Ongoing Process

The beauty of mindfulness lies in its simplicity. It is not something we need to strive for or achieve; rather, it is something we cultivate moment by moment. Each time we return to the present, we engage in the process of mindfulness. It is not about reaching a final goal or attaining perfection, but about continually showing up for ourselves with awareness, presence, and intention.

In this sense, mindfulness is a process of becoming. It is an ongoing unfolding, a journey that evolves as we deepen our practice and understanding. The more we practice mindfulness, the more we come to understand the interconnectedness of all things, and the more we learn to navigate life with grace and presence. It is a process that invites us to live with purpose and authenticity, to be fully present in each moment, and to approach life with a sense of curiosity and wonder.

Through mindfulness, we learn to appreciate the richness of our experiences, both the joys and the challenges. It helps us to embrace life as it is, without judgment or expectation. In doing so, we create the space for transformation and growth. Each moment of mindfulness becomes an opportunity to let go of old patterns and make more intentional choices. It is a practice that invites us to live fully and authentically, in alignment with our deepest values and aspirations.

Mindfulness, then, is not something that we achieve once and for all. It is a continuous, ongoing practice that evolves as we do. And in this practice, we find the freedom to live more fully, more consciously, and with greater purpose.